The Clay Disciples

by

Cano Graham

With my deepest respect and admiration, a special and lasting thank you goes to Dick and Betty Liddell of Norman, Oklahoma. Only with their faith and material assistance has this book been completed.

I also offer my eternal love and gratitude to those once in a lifetime friends in Tecopa Hot Springs, California, who so generously gave their talents, energy and hearts to our Crystal Cross Therapeutic Clay Center, and the movement of Clay Therapy: Ruthie Badame, Sylvia Burton, Art and Luella Babbitt, Mori Rubenstein, Beulah Rosenberg, Joyce Lassos, and Curt Hibdon

For You With Love

by Louis Untermeyer

Love is the whisper of earth,
when the stars pale
and the dawn winds hail
a new day's birth.

The laughing abandon,
the shining glee
of the fountain's leap
and the headlong sweep of the sea.
Love is the memory that time can't kill;
the cherished tune gay and absurd
and the music unheard.

The silence, that trembles,
and seems to fill the heart
when the song of a bird is still.

Love is God's plenty;
an endless measure of gifts
that descend in sun and shower,
on mountain and plain,
the quickening rain
and the storied treasure
at the rainbow's end.

Love is the coming alive
of a golden bush that can't wait for Spring
blossoms that bring joy to the day
and honey to the hive.
The call of the hills
and the answering ocean,
when everything is a maze
and a blaze of color and motion,
torrents of wonder of waves
and wings and the whole sky sings.

But first and last;
time present,
time future,
time past,
past all belief and thinking of
earth beneath and heaven above;
beginning and ending
forever new.
Love is you.

With love for all of you,
    Cano Graham

Forward

Recall the face of the poorest and weakest man who you may have seen, and ask yourself if the step you contemplate is going to be of any use to him.   Gandhi

You will find this a simple book to understand.

I don't consider myself a polished writer, nor am I a physician. Those issues aside, I have had an extraordinary opportunity to explore firsthand the revered healing power of the ancient substance called clay. My motives come not from wanting to write, but rather because something desperately needs to be said.

The existing and future circumstance of our health care system dictates that each person assumes the ultimate responsibility for his or her own well-being. Within our nation's alternative medicine movement, many of us have our own primary vehicle. We call ourselves *The Clay Disciples*.

Introduction

Someday 1972

We have more ability than will power, and it is more often an excuse to ourselves that we imagine that things are impossible.

Francois De La Rochefoucauld

At 40 years old, I found myself disappointed, depressed, frightened and angry. Eighteen months of constant, piercing back and sciatic pain, which included seventeen physicians, ten days in a V.A. hospital, 18-24 aspirins and 6-8 Darvons every day, had left me nearly bankrupt in every department of my life. I went on a desperate search for someone, anyone, who could help me.

I woke up at three or four a.m. because of paralyzing spasms. Like an addict, I fumbled for my glass of water and washed down a few of the ever-present Darvons to relax the grip of pain. After this routine, I pulled myself out of bed, shuffled zombie-style around the apartment to loosen the trauma on my whole body, and eventually collapsed back into bed for some precious rest. Each day I woke in a panic knowing that I faced another day of pain. I saw no end in sight.

How true the quote of St. Augustine of Hippo, "The greatest evil is physical pain." I prayed to the Power that if I could simply be made pain free, I would do something meaningful with my life. As I wrote *The Clay Disciples* I often reflected on that covenant.

11

Early November 1972 was overcast in the Los Angeles, California basin, and found me deteriorating physically and emotionally. I had been steered to a physician in Fullerton, not too far from beautiful Carbon Canyon, where I lived.

After I had related again, for what seemed like the hundredth time, the situation I was in, I pleaded as only a person in pain can plead. "Do you think you can help me, Doc?"

A reassuring smile broke his aloof demeanor, as he considered the answer. He delivered his rhetoric in a fatherly fashion, soaked with a bland, patronizing attitude. He'd obviously played this scene often, and it came up too stale, too flat, too mushy, and far, far too familiar.

Then he uttered the timeless cliché, which is always delivered as if in the name of all humanity. "Mr. Graham, if I didn't think I could help you, I wouldn't take you as a patient."

The words "take you" stuck in my head and I cratered a bit because I had heard that refrain before, several times, many times in fact. All those physicians who came before had said something akin to, "If I didn't think I could help you..." The words flashed like a strobe light before me.

My mind was rolling those scenes of disappointment when I recalled an experience I'd had just that morning in my bank. I had unexpectedly coughed, and a pain like a massive electric shock instantly threw me to the cold terrazzo floor. As I lay stunned, flat on my back, a nice little old lady asked, "Are you alright, dear?"

I didn't even remember going down.

I sat directly in front of the doctor, reliving the morning's experience when I had been without energy or hope.

The doctor repeated, "Sir? Sir? Mr. Graham?"

I sort of went blank as I heard him utter again, "If I didn't think I could help you..."

I quit listening. A cold voice I almost didn't recognize slipped from my throat. "Does that mean if you can't help me, then I don't have to pay you?"

The question hung like acrid smoke in a garbage dump. I saw him freeze. Ever so slightly, his eyes squinted, as if peering through a thick fog. The moment broke with a slight clearing of his throat. Then as if a decision had been reached, with forefinger and thumb, he cleaned invisible crumbs from the corners of his mouth. His head swayed in an unconscious and foolish manner. This man had a definite conflict of interest in progress. His conscience and the status quo were not on the same page.

He flinched. "Well, no. I mean that there will be...there must be my fees."

First, I sensed mere deception, then overt betrayal by the establishment. I lashed back vehemently. "For what? You just said you wouldn't take me as a patient if you didn't think you could help me! Just what *are* you saying? Tell me why in hell I should pay you for bad judgment?"

He reminded me of a kid with his hand caught in the cookie jar. "If you were a TV repairman I wouldn't pay unless you fixed my television. If you were a mechanic, you'd have to fix the car or you wouldn't get paid. It seems that in this world we all sell either a service or a product, and we don't get paid until we deliver either the product or the service! So, why in God's name should I pay you anything unless you can do what you say you can do, and that is help me! Get me out of pain or you don't get a dime!"

I stood shaking. I had snapped. I screamed, "Why? Why? Why?"

The nurse opened the door. The doctor glanced at her and then back at me. In front of her, he took the offensive with a condescending attitude. "Sir, I believe you're upset."

I yelled back. "Upset? You ass! I'm in pain! Don't you understand? *P-A-I-N! Twenty-four hours a day, P-A-I-N!* Either take me as a patient, or not, but enough of your double talk! You get paid for results, not your sanctimonious bullshit! Got it?"

He retreated into that damn routine of swaying again, which made me feel as if it were only his options he was concerned with, certainly not mine.

An eerie silence fell over the room. I was weak, completely drained of energy. I sat, slumped and powerless, supporting my head in my hands. I had nothing left.

I whispered, "It's not right. It's just not fair. The system is wrong." I raised my eyes and said, "No one should pay hard-earned money if the treatment doesn't work. Someday it's gonna be different. Someday."

I brushed the naïve plea aside with an unforgiving wave of my hand. I felt like a child cheated at a carnival. I rose and shuffled to the door.

I sensed the physician identified with me, yet he stood mute.

Then in the most sincere and compassionate voice, the nurse said, "I'm sorry, Mr. Graham."

I believe she meant well, and that she also really understood. She smiled slightly and added, "Someday."

Chapter 1

A fresh breeze

Destiny grants us our wishes to give us something beyond our wishes.   Johann Wolfgang Von Goethe

New Year's Eve 1986, 6:00 P.M.
Eva Graham's home
Chino, California

For the past several years, mom and I had spent the holidays together, whether she lived in Oklahoma, Texas, or Nevada. We enjoyed the same New Year's ritual every year. We had some eggnog and she'd turn in. I'd take a long walk and get to bed by 10:00 p.m. We'd get up early and I'd take a meditative first run of the year while she fixed a special breakfast for us. Then we'd watch the parades and football games all day long. Watching her happiness gave me the greatest joy. That little routine lasted for twenty years. Mother, Joyce Lassos, a charming and reserved 47 year-old yoga instructor, and I sat down to our evening dinner.

As I helped myself to a baked potato, I asked mother, "Hey, Mom, did you wash these potatoes?"

Joyce looked at me, then at mom, and back at her potato, with the odd expression as if to say "Why did he ask that?"

Mom didn't let Joyce hang too long on the question, and as I seriously examined my potato, mom broke the spell by laughing and saying, "Oh Cano, stop that!" Then she answered in a singsong, did-it-a-million-times manner, "Yes, I washed the potatoes."

To make sense of the scene for our new friend, Mom turned to her and continued. "Dear, don't pay any attention to him. He's been doing that since he was a little boy."

Relieved, Joyce said, "Well, I wondered."

Mom patted her hand. "I took Cano with me to dig potatoes when he was four years old. The next day I fixed baked potatoes, and Cano asked, 'Momma, did you wash these potatoes?' He was serious because he had spent the day digging potatoes out of the dirt. I told him, 'Yes honey, Momma washed the potatoes.' Then he said, 'Well, that's good.'"

I laughed at the memory.

"After that digging experience, he always asked that question, until he was around ten years old or so, in front of friends, anywhere. After that it was just a game."

Joyce enjoyed mom's explanation of the ritual. The dinner went well, and we moved to the front room when mom said, "Cano, what's on your mind? Seems like you're thinking about something."

I smiled, went over to where she sat and kissed her forehead. "You know your third son, don't you honey? Well, could be. Do you two care for some more champagne?"

Mom winked at Joyce. "We were waiting for you to ask." And then, so curious she could hardly stand it, she said, "What is it? Something's been on your mind the past few days. You're thinking about something."

Mom always fancied herself a bit psychic, and there were times when she made us all wonder.

"Yeah, Mom, you're right. Something's on my mind. Say how'd you two like to go to the desert for a New Year's Eve party then stay there for tomorrow?"

"Nope, not me." She held her glass out for a refill.

I knew Mom wouldn't care to go.

"This year I'd just like to enjoy the day alone." She squinted her eyes after puckering her lips. "I have a hunch that this idea of going to the desert didn't just happen. Joyce, watch him. Something's going on between his ears." We all laughed at mother's critique of the moment.

She was right and I asked, "You don't mind being alone?"

She said, "Joyce, he knows better than that. He knows that when I'm alone I'm not lonely. Not if I've got something to do, and I know where my boys are. Tomorrow I've got a whole pile of alterations I can work on while I watch the games." She pointed at me. "Besides, you, mister! You have something on your mind!"

Joyce felt caught in the crossfire. While waving her glass at me for a refill she said to Mom, "Come on Eva, come with us. Please? Pretty please?" The women in my life adored mother because she always took their side of any issue.

Mom said, "No! No! I'll be just fine here. I want to catch the parades and all. I wouldn't think of it, but you'd better be ready for anything. It's a big desert."

Concerned, Joyce asked, "Cano, what are we going to do? Eva, what's he up to? What's going on?"

Mom was having fun with Joyce's curiosity and whispered, "He acts like he doesn't know where he's going, but he does. His path is to stay off the trail. It's always been that way. Once we found him a mile-and-a-half from home, walking along a country road when he was only eighteen months old! Watch him. And you two have fun."

I was antsy. Earlier that day I had fueled, washed, and waxed my 1957 Pontiac Chieftain, a beautiful, off-white and turquoise two-door hardtop, making it the spiffiest thing on the road. The car had so much chrome it bordered on sinful. We threw some things in a suitcase, and I said, "Okay, Mom, we're outta here. I'll call you tomorrow afternoon."

Saying, "Please drive careful," Mom handed Joyce a sack. "There's some fruit and things for later on and maybe tomorrow. Make him drive slow."

Joyce hugged and kissed Mom. "Don't worry, I will. Thanks a bunch for the afternoon and a great dinner. It was so special."

We headed east on the Pomona Freeway. You can find fun in any trip particularly when you're not really sure what's ahead, and you stay loose. Joyce sat close and the thought of going to Palm Springs caused her affection to increase.

When we got to the interchange where Interstate 15 North crosses the Pomona Freeway going east, I moved to the right lane, and onto the I-15 heading north toward Las Vegas.

"What are you doing? Where are you going? Palm Springs is straight ahead! You said we were going to the desert!"

"Yep, you're right on one count. We are going to the desert, but not to Palm Springs."

"But Palm Springs is the desert!"

"Right, but not the only place in the desert!"

She moved to the far right of the seat now, and said, "What desert are we going to?"

Enjoying the moment, I said, "Have you ever heard of Death Valley?"

She turned full around, pretended choking, and with the most bewildered look exclaimed, "Death Valley! What in the world are we going to do in Death Valley?"

This was getting better by the minute. I reached into the back seat and got a big bottle of Bailey's Irish Cream and handed it to her. "Would you mind opening this? It's full of goodness."

"Fine. But, Death Valley?"

"Well, it's not actually *in* Death Valley. It's a place called Tecopa Hot Springs."

She mumbled, "Eva said to watch out, that you were thinking about something. Cano! Where is Teacup, whatever the name is, Hot Springs? I'm dressed for Palm Springs!"

18

We cruised up the Cajón Pass and left the Los Angeles basin behind. As we got close to Victorville, Joyce still hadn't mellowed much. She kept saying, "Eva tried to tell me, Oh, great!" Then punctuated her displeasure. "I've got to use the bathroom."

"Fine. No problem. I'll get us some coffee for the Bailey's while you go. Before too long I've got another nice treat that you're going to love."

"Just let me find a restroom! I don't need any more of your surprises!" Still talking to herself she said, "Eva told me! Darn! What a New Year's Eve party this is!"

Presently, Joyce trotted back and jumped in the car. She faked a shiver, and said, "It's cold up here! Where are you taking me?"

I raised a devilish eyebrow and replied like the villain in a melodrama, "Away, my dear, away!"

She fell back in the seat and moaned, "Oh my God. Eva told me."

At 10:30 that night, we passed Barstow, heading for Baker. Joyce forgot her pretended anger and spun the radio dial, looking for some music.

"Hey, Lady, about ready for the other surprise?"

Her eyes rolled and she looked at me as if to say, "What did I do to deserve this?"

Before her eyes quit rolling, an idea popped and Joyce's attitude changed from mock displeasure to full out positive. She taunted me. "Mister G., you got me on the potatoes and dragging me to Death Valley, but now it's my turn." She snickered playfully.

I didn't have a clue where this was going, but I took a sip of Baileys, and grinned at her new energy. "Okay my little fireball, what's up?"

She twisted around and in two seconds her pretty derriere

poked up in the air as she leaned over the seat searching through her overnight bag. "Alright, Mister-likes-surprises-Graham, I'll tell you what's up. It's *you*! You're going to be *up*." Then she found her treasure. "Yes. I have one!!"

"One what?"

"Question for you, sir: Do you ever smoke?"

"No, quit a long time ago."

"Silly, I'm talking about pot."

"Pot? Oh I have, but not too often. Pretty much stopped when I started my acting career. Is that grass?"

"Sure is. Are you chicken or will you join me? I know it's illegal, but it's just *one*."

"Well! I didn't know you indulged."

Joyce bobbed her head side to side, and enjoyed taking the offense. "Just on special occasions, and this night certainly qualifies. Will you?"

"Here? Now?"

"Right now, Mister-smarty-pants Graham."

I laughed and conceded. "I must say, you do have a way with words. Sure, I'm game for a toke or two. You got me."

"Oh good! This will be a hoot. I'm going to love seeing you high."

She was cute and classy.

In a few minutes we were warm, cozy, and the Chieftain cruised as if thoroughly enjoying having my guest along, and almost as if it knew where we were going. Joyce caught a little buzz, enough for her to ask some questions she ordinarily wouldn't ask, and I was mellow enough to answer what I would have normally avoided.

We were having a ball. We turned north at Baker on Highway 127, heading to Death Valley and it was such a relief to be off the freeway! We didn't see another car on the road. I cranked up the radio and we sang along with Kenny Rogers and Dolly Parton.

Islands in the stream,
that's what we are,
nothing in between,
how can we be wrong,
sail away with me to another world,
and we'll rely on each other uh huh…
from one lover to another uh huh…

We were like kids on a lark.

Ten minutes outside of Baker, I let the Chieftain roll to a stop. We stepped out into a fabulous, velvety black, utterly silent, desert night. The crisp air, brilliant sky, and the isolation cast their own magic. Joyce and I were dwarfed by the majesty of our moment. We just stood there with our arms around each other.

She spoke softly. "Oh my! I had no idea."

I nodded my head in awe. "Yep Baby, *this* is the other treat."

"Cano, it's wonderful! I'm sorry I acted so. I didn't know."

"Hey, no problem. You're a great sport." I kissed her cheek. "Yes, Yes, it is magnificent."

After a few minutes we started to roll again. The chilly air invigorated us but we didn't realize how much until back in the warm car, and on the road. Chilled, Joyce snuggled close.

As we sipped some Bailey's, Joyce said, "You know Cano, I read an article about you before we met."

"You did? What article?"

"The article in the *Santa Ana Register* on Mother's Day. The one about you doing the research on The Greeter in Laguna Beach. Was it 1980, or 81?"

"Right now I don't have a solid answer for good morning. I'm not sure about the date. Whoa! I think I'm a bit high!"

"Good! This is fun. I also wondered, how did it all start?"

I turned the radio down. "The Greeter? I wanted a project to do, a play or film, and he was such an unusual character I realized his story would be…"

Joyce interrupted. "No sweetheart, I mean how did you start your career? Eva told me that you were 45 when you started. Cano, are you listening to me?"

"Yeah, babe, I'm listening. I was, thinking, you wanna know how my career happened? Okay, a lot of story, just real quick, because I don't want to start tripping on this."

Joyce laughed. "I think maybe you already are." She sounded almost timid when she held up the joint. "Do you want anymore of this?"

"No. I'm good to go, but you go ahead."

Joyce shook her head. "No, I'm fine too."

I got to thinking about way back when.

She said, "Cano? Hello? Are you going to talk to me?"

"Oh yeah. Sure. Sorry, I was drifting."

She kissed me on the cheek, smiled, and said, "I know, but talk to me."

"Alright, here goes. Nice and quick. I wanted to be an actor since I was twelve or thirteen years old."

"Are you kidding? Why did you wait so long?"

I shrugged, "I was one of the Graham Boys, supposed to be like my brother Paul, you know, all-State football and basketball. He was my idol! In my hometown, I didn't think they'd ever approve of me being an actor. I mean after all, actors, singers, and piano players were all sissies. Acting would have been against my image!"

"Your image?"

We laughed again. "Baby, if you'd been from Shawnee, Oklahoma in the 40s and 50s, you'd damn well know what I'm talking about."

She appeared to be enjoying the confession.

"Hell, I was jumping out of airplanes as an eighteen-year old kid in the Paratroopers, just to prove how tough I was, or rather to prove to *them* how tough I wanted them to think I was."

She came closer, kissed me on the cheek and half whispered,

"Since you were twelve?"

"That's right. Then one day I moved, didn't tell a soul, and started my career as an actor."

"You didn't tell anyone? You just did it? Didn't you tell Eva, or your brother or someone?"

"Nope, no one. It was just too private. I can't explain why, I just didn't want anyone to know."

I began to reflect on the work I'd done as an actor. Joyce rested her head in my lap and closed her eyes. I thought that maybe she had fallen asleep. I relived the first exciting day at the Strasberg Institute in Hollywood, when I experienced a sensation similar to going home.

"Hey Joyce, are you awake?"

She patted my leg. "Yes, I'm awake. Go ahead."

"Well, you know how close mother and I are?"

"Yes, it's fun to see you two together. She loves you so. Is this about her?"

"Actually, there are two different stories. They'll take a few minutes. Would you rather nap awhile?"

"C'mon, Cano, tell me now. I'm just resting my eyes. I love your stories about her. Go ahead."

I stroked her hair. "So, like I said, I've wanted to act since I was a little boy. Well, like I said, not one person knew what I was doing. Not one!"

"You mean you just dropped out completely? What did you tell your friends?"

"Nothing! I broke free. I felt brand new, and I'd let 'em know when I was ready for them to see my work. I wasn't interested in talking about the issue. I was doing it."

"Well, I'd been at the Institute for only two weeks and was asked to play the lead in a production because some actor got a job. Anyway, now get this Joyce, I'm only forty-five minutes before opening in my first play, I spotted the pay telephone next to a water fountain backstage. Just as I started my preparation work, I impulsively picked up the phone and called mom."

"You must have been excited."

"Well, yes I was. Actually, it was the wrong time to call, so close to curtain time. I just did it before I really thought much about it.

"After some small talk, she wanted to know what I was doing. I wasn't about to discuss my acting career, so I put her off by saying, 'not much, same ole thing. Then Mom came up with a strange sort of question. She asked,

'Are you starting any new projects? Or doing anything different?'

"When she asked me such a curious question, I sort of got a queasy feeling in the pit of my stomach. I casually replied, "Oh, I've been toying with an idea, but nothing for sure."

Mom pressed me.

"Honey, I don't want to go into it. It's nothing. Well, not exactly nothing, sort of a hobby."

"Please tell me," she begged.

"Come on Mom, I don't want to waste time talking about something that's nothing."

Mom laughed. "Can I guess?"

"Joyce, here I was forty minutes from opening my *first* play! Like it was time to start my preparation work!"

"What did you do?"

"Do? Jesus! I just rolled my eyes back, chuckled at the situation and said, 'Sure honey, you can guess.' I mean, Joyce, I was seriously busting up inside and thinking, 'Here I am, backstage 2000 miles away, about to go on stage at the Strasberg Institute, and no one, including my closest friends, know what I'm doing, and my little momma wants to guess! Yeah right! Gimme a break! Was this too much or what?"

"What happened?"

"The next thing I know Mom said, 'Be right back.' I said, 'Wait a minute, where ya going?' Mom replied, 'I've got a note on my bed stand, you know I keep track of all dreams.' I said, 'Okay,'" and stepped aside to get a sip of water while she left the phone.

"Well, she came back and started reading from her dream book. 'No, that's not it. No. Oh, it was just a couple of weeks ago. Here it is! I've got it! Honey, now don't laugh, but has this thing you're doing got anything to do with drama or movies? Kind of like acting, you know, like acting on stage on front of people?"

Joyce sat bolt upright. "She what? Cano, do you mean that Eva dreamed of you acting?"

I nodded and sipped Bailey's at the same time. "It knocked me out. I remember feeling as if I had electricity in my head."

"What'd you do?"

"All I could say was, 'Mom what in the world would make you think such a thing?"

Mom replied, "I can't imagine. They were just dreams, *but so real*. I've had several since. Even last night again, real clear. I can remember it, isn't this strange? This whole thing started on October 12th. I suppose it's harmless enough. Does that day mean anything to you Cano? Cano, are you there? Honey is something wrong?"

"It was unbelievable, too much. I mean, for a few seconds I couldn't respond. I felt flush, like a fever had swept over me-or something! Joyce, October 12, 1977 was the day that I began my acting career at the Strasberg Institute in Los Angeles."

"Why haven't you told me about this before?"

"Why? Hell, it'll take a little time to tell everything about her. Some things you just don't walk around talking about. It's something though, huh?"

"Unreal! This connection between you and Eva is remarkable."

"You know I never knew until the past couple of years, but Mom told me some things about her personal life that my brothers never knew. I know they didn't. She told me I was her and Dad's favorite, and in fact she said that I was planned. Isn't that something? To be planned?"

We were both silent-lost in thought. All the windows were down, her blonde hair was flying, and the Chief was rolling. We were oblivious to the icy wind.

After a minute or so, Joyce broke the spell. "I think it's wonderful," and she scooted closer for warmth.

C８ C８ C８

My mind drifted to the wonderful years I shared with Lorrie Hull, my acting coach and roommate, who directed much of my acting work. I relived the thrill of beginning my days as an actor. I loved running to the top of Mulholland Drive above the Hollywood Bowl and out onto a bluff overlooking Hollywood and L.A. Then with my arms raised in victory, I yelled at the top of my lungs, knowing that no one could hear me. I screamed my dream.

"My name is Cano, and I'm an actooooooorrrr!"

With that ritual completed, I'd jog down through the hills to our apartment and begin my day.

As the Chief rolled on and Joyce slept, I thought back to when I had returned from the film in Mexico, knowing it was time to take the hair and beard off. The hair and beard had been fun. I'd done a lot of work and completed my research on The Greeter, but it had also cost me in terms of jobs as a contemporary actor.

I had no idea the memories that replayed in my brain were in fact my Swan Song as an actor.

My commercial agents said, "Now's your time, Cano. The hair and beard have got to come off. You could go on an interview everyday, but not unless you're contemporary. You've already lost two major jobs because you wouldn't cut your hair."

I agreed. "Okay. Lots of people in town don't know me any other way, casting agents and so forth. I know it's time to do it, but give me a couple of months. I want to have some fun with it. I've got the germ of an idea. My mom has her 83rd birthday coming up in a couple of months and I'm thinking of having a few friends get together and make a surprise party out of cutting my hair. Something like that anyway."

They looked at each other with the blankest stares I'd ever seen.

I tried to defend my position. "Hey, I've got an idea! Let me play with it, okay?"

"Play with it hell! You're costing yourself money. You just lost a job that most of our clients would give their right arms for. Look at this! A $17,000 contract to do Marlboro commercials in Germany. This isn't chopped liver, Cano."

"All right guys, all right. I'll see ya in a couple of months. I want to chew on my idea for a while. I'd like to figure an interesting way to reintroduce myself to the industry. Something else you need to know. You may think I'm kidding, but I'm not. I didn't turn that contract down because I didn't want to cut my hair. I wouldn't do a nicotine commercial for $117,000! See ya at my party."

It took a few weeks for the whole idea to gel. I had three months to draw it all together. I set the date of March 7, 1983 to pull it off.

I decided to make the night a full evening of entertainment. The basic idea was even more interesting than I had originally thought. The program for the evening included a full sit-down dinner before I performed the wonderful one-hour play *The Dirty Old Man*. Then I'd have a barber cut my long hair and shave my beard on stage. I then intended to go backstage, change from my old clothes costume, finish cleaning up, and in approximately twenty minutes, come back on stage in a nice three-piece suit as a new man.

During the change, I planned to have some live music playing to fill the time. After twenty minutes, the MC would call mother up on stage to generally discuss the evening, which would lead to asking Mom how old she was. I knew she'd respond by saying she'd just had her eighty-third birthday.

At that point I'd emerge from backstage carrying a birthday cake loaded with eighty-three blazing candles, and all one hundred and sixty-five guests would sing, "Happy Birthday, Dear Eva!" Oh, yes, I would pull off the Great Surprise Party Caper.

The plan had a problem, though. By all rights, it had far too many moving parts to make it work. Finally, however, I had drawn it all together, and it had the potential for a fine evening, I still had my concerns though because in theater, the difference between potential and reality can be chaos. I had to find a director, a stage manager, and actors to do the play. Plus I wanted to have some quality entertainment for the twenty-minute break.

I had to have invitations designed and printed. I decided to charge $7.50 per person for the dinner and the evening of entertainment, to cover basic costs. I asked John Randolf, the great actor and founder of the Ensemble Theatre Group, to which I belonged, to act as my director. Our rehearsals had gone well, and we were close to ready.

While some friends discussed the unusual and fun nature of the evening, I threw out the question of who I could get, or what I could get, without spending any more money, to act as entertainment during the break. In other words, who would be right, and free?

This fellow I'd only known for about a year said, "Cano, I think you need a singer. One that your audience, and especially your mom would enjoy. Someone who could bring his own piano accompanist, and cost you nothing!"

"Right. Sure, Tony. But who?"

I was having this conversation with one of the truly great singing stars since the Golden Era of Hollywood. His signature song was the immortal, "Begin the Beguine." The fabulous, incomparable Tony Martin playfully scratched his chin as though trying to solve the problem when he slyly let his idea out. "Cano, I feel that there's only one guy that can really fill the bill."

"Yeah, Tony, who?"

That handsome face smiled. "Obviously me!"

ଓ ଓ ଓ

When March 7th arrived I felt good but apprehensive about bringing it all together. I cut all of the foliage for the set out of the Hollywood Hills early in the morning, then hauled everything downtown in my old '67 Ford pickup, to the legendary Embassy Theater for the stage. By four p.m. exhausted but feeling great, I felt ready.

My brother had brought mom down from Las Vegas, Nevada. We had a packed house, and the staff served a wonderful dinner right on time. I wasn't aware that some friends from the Ensemble Theatre Group had hurriedly set up a video camera to capture the moment. But even they didn't know the sound wasn't working until the last fifteen minutes of the evening.

Bob Weiss, President of the Author's Club of America and a dear friend of mine, served as master of ceremonies and did a terrific job of running the show. The dinner went just as planned, and high energy charged the air.

The curtains opened to a beautiful set depicting a wooded clearing, overlooking the ocean in Northern California. The actors, D.B. Brown, Shelley Green, and I playing the lead, performed. We nailed it! The audience loved it.

After the play ended, I took center stage and the crowd got a big kick out of watching the bulk of five years of hair and beard shorn away. . With most of the hair gone, I retreated backstage to finish cleaning up. I changed into a suit and prepared to go back on stage with the huge birthday cake just as Tony was leading the audience in a surprise chorus of "Happy Birthday."

Tony was terrific. It was easy to see why he'd been a star for forty years. After twenty minutes, he called mother on stage. She was radiant, and the only person in the room who wasn't in on the surprise party!

The audience, fully aware of what the evening was about, was anxious to meet mom. Tony got her relaxed and they started talking. She stole the show and the audience fell in love with her. Mom thought it was just terrible that Tony Martin hadn't asked for payment. Then the audience, which by now included all the busboys and cooks from the kitchen, began to sing "Happy Birthday, dear Eva."

I didn't plan on the next step working so well, but when I came back onstage, the only person in the entire room who couldn't see me holding the birthday cake with eighty-three candles was mother. Tony had her turned so that I could come up behind her, and with the last few words of the song being sung, I yelled, "Mom!"

She turned around and realized that someone was holding this big, candle-lit cake and the audience wanted her to blow out the candles! Well, eighty-three candles took a lot of blowing. She took a deep breath and started blowing from left to right. Few could see, but as she started this Herculean effort, I silently blew hard from right to left.

This impulsive act created a mini-whirlwind of sorts. Swoosh! From the audience, it appeared that mom had blown out all eighty-three candles in one magnificent moment! The audience erupted with wild applause. She was so used to me with the long hair and beard and so excited, that Mom didn't recognize me until I set the cake down! The audience went nuts!

When the evening came to a close, I looked around the room and realized that the evening had been even more magical than I ever conceived. I couldn't find mother. Finally, I found her in a small anteroom, sitting in one of those high-backed, throne-like wicker chairs. She was dressed beautifully that night in a long black floor-length full skirt, and a white blouse with a frill of lace around the collar that went up high on her neck. Sitting in that high-backed chair, she looked splendid.

"Honey, I couldn't find you. What are you doing?"

She smiled and said something unlike anything I'd ever heard her say before. "Honey, come and sit down with me for just a minute."

She took my hand, and in the sweetest moment of my life said, "Honey, I want you to know that today has been the single best day of my life."

No one has ever said anything to me that has meant as much. In a split second, I realized she had lived 83 years, had literally thousands of wonderful days, and a sack full of great memories, yet she said this had been the best night of her life.

I cracked the wing-window of the Chief, took a deep breath and thought, "Me too, Mom. The best night of my life'.

Out of nowhere, Joyce asked, "Are you hungry?"

"Lady, I've got a fierce case of the munchies right now!"

"Me too. Oh, I'd love some of that pie Eva made!"

"Can't help you there, but check out the sack of stuff Mom gave us. She always puts more in than you can eat."

My usually demure yoga instructor dove into the sack like an eight-year-old going after Halloween goodies. "Yeow! Yes! Oreo cookies!" She acted like a street beggar. "Do you have any ice cream mister? *Please?"*

We busted out laughing while we stuffed Oreo cookies into our mouths. We acted like a couple of teenagers on a lark. Finally we settled down, found some soft rock, and cruised along with no traffic at 40 mph.

"This is too much," Joyce said and laid down on the seat with her head in my lap. Then in her very feminine manner, "I'm glad we didn't go to Palm Springs. This is neat!"

"Well said, Miss J, this is fun and we've got a couple of days to go."

Joyce seemed pleased. She pinched me and said, "Yummy!"

Ⅎ Ⅎ Ⅎ

The Chief floated across the rolling desert like a fancy powerboat gliding over gentle swells.

"Cano?"

"What?" I knew a question was coming.

"How'd you start? Why?"

"How'd I start what? Why what?"

She said, "The 'biz' I overheard you call it your 'biz.' I'm sorry, I shouldn't have asked."

I seldom discussed my illegal business, my biz, even with good friends who had a fair idea of where my money came from. In this case, however, the Holiday Spirit, the herb, plus our comfort level all conspired to turn me on.

"My biz? Well, it just sort of happened. I mean, I made what at first I thought of as an innocent move." I glanced at her. "Well, I don't know how innocent, but I loaned a friend a few hundred dollars. He said he'd pay me back over the weekend, with big interest." I glanced at her again. "Okay, I knew he wasn't investing in the stock market. Although he didn't say he was selling grass." I laughed, "By the way, that's called rationalizing.

"Anyway, I started loaning him money on a regular basis, and soon our business arrangement turned into a full-blown operation to sell pot. So now you know, but frankly I didn't intend to be so, shall we say, active."

Joyce yawned. "That's not too exciting." She changed the subject. "How far do we have to go?"

I stroked her hair. "Not far, maybe fifteen or twenty miles. We'll be there in half an hour."

She squeezed my leg. "Oh, good! Wake me up when we get there." She had a smile in her voice when she said, "Eva was right. You do have a reason for coming up here. You do have something on your mind."

"Yes, I do, and you'll see it soon enough."

I knew Joyce was pleased as she patted my leg. I let her doze off. I began thinking of a casual conversation at a Christmas party I had attended the previous week. Had it only been a week ago?

My brother, Dr. Frank Graham, and two of his colleagues were vigorously discussing the virtues and pitfalls of the medical field in general, and the pharmaceutical field in particular, and where it was heading in the next few years. During that candid conversation, the spark of an idea, which had been smoldering for some time burst into flame. The fire ignited because I frankly didn't care much for the overall attitude of those young physicians, or for the forecast they so arrogantly predicted. Dr. Frank, my younger brother by eighteen months, watched me react to the young physician's conventional point of view. He winked, and nodded his head for us to go outside.

I thought he wanted to execute our life-long ritual. When we were kids we had a daily contest to see who could pee the furthest, but tonight we decided to forego the event. He said, "Bud, how'd you like to take a walk?"

That sounded fine to me because I had tired of all the talk inside. I said, "Good. Let's go. What's up?"

"Hey big bro' you tell me. What's going on?"

I missed his meaning, "About what?"

He started to explain what I thought wasn't so obvious. "I've never heard you ask so many pointed questions. Are you thinking about buying a medical clinic or something?"

"It showed that much, huh?"

"Sho' did, bro', sho' did."

"Well," I said, "I'm considering the subject. I'm just not sure of the direction to go, or what I want to do, but frankly, after listening to those two guys, man, I'm ready for something."

They had jolted me into realizing that the time was ripe to move forward with my idea for a Holistic Center.

I had made the decision to open a small spa somewhere, not too big, just enough to get started, and then I'd add services as I gained knowledge and recognized needs. A live-in manager could handle day-to-day activities while I aggressively continued my acting career.

At that moment we hit the crest of a hill and I could see the lights of Tecopa Hot Springs.

I brushed the hair from Joyce's face and whispered, "Helloooo, we're here."

She sat up, half-asleep, then laid her head on my shoulder. "What time is it?"

I glanced at the car clock. "Happy New Year, girl! It's 1987!"

We rolled into Tecopa Hot Springs at about 12:45. "This is it? Doesn't look like much but a bunch of RVs," she said.

Looking everywhere at once I said, "You know what, I've only been here one time. I had a problem with my back in '84 while in Death Valley. I came here for the hot mineral water, and it worked! Hey, sleepyhead, let's cruise all over this place."

With closed eyes, she mumbled, "Not much here, shouldn't take too long."

I was excited. "I love it! This is like a big canvas to paint on. Vegas is just over an hour away; Death Valley, less than an hour. We have L.A. less than four hours away, and Baker and I-15 are less than an hour. Look at this! Only one stop sign!"

"Cano, as slow as you're driving it'll be morning before we get to sleep. You *really* do like the place!"

"I don't have to copy anything here. I can create something and do it my way!"

She got a kick out of watching me so turned on by the funky little community. Then she reverted to the little beggar role and said, "Mr. Graham, I'm tired. Have you made up your mind?"

"About what?"

"About where we're going to stay?"

I leaned over and kissed her cheek. "Yes ma'am, I have, and I've just made another decision too. I'll tell you about that one tomorrow."

I had decided where to stay, but more important, I pretty much knew the spot I wanted to buy—a small motel on high ground with only a few rooms, but it had hot baths and the only hot mineral water swimming pool in town.

I checked us in and unpacked the car. We threw on robes and headed straight for the enclosed hot water swimming pool, a relaxing finish to our evening.

We slept late on New Year's Day, and after a breakfast at the Miner's Diner in Tecopa, we enjoyed a beer at the infamous Snake Pit.

About one o'clock in the afternoon, we returned, and I bought the place that went by the exotic name of Ali Baba's, an absolute wreck on three acres, but I loved it!

Strange how things work out. The dream of my life, my acting career, would soon be subordinated by the twisting hands of fate. Step by step I had been guided to Tecopa Hot Springs and the paramount chapter of my life, to submerge myself in the discipline of using clay therapeutically. Exciting new winds had begun to swirl.

Chapter 2

Tecopa, Tecopa Hot Springs, California

The ornaments of a house are the friends who frequent it.
Ralph Waldo Emerson

By the 1930s, 40s, and 50s, Tecopa, California had grown into a major rail center, with tons of borax passing through from Death Valley to Barstow, California. Home to 4,000 robust citizens, chief among them miners and their families, who worked the many major talc, lead, and silver mines in the immediate vicinity.

The eventual closing of these mines gutted Tecopa in a devastating implosion, leaving no one in charge, no employer, or payroll. They did have a church, a post office, a small store, a café, a bar, a few small vacant buildings, and a fine reservoir of folks who loved their oasis and refused to give up and head for town.

The Shoshone Indians originally inhabited this land and utilized the natural healing springs for a thousand years or more before the settlers found the healing mud the Indians called *Eewah-kee*, the earth that heals.

Forty years ago, Inyo County, operating in agreement with the Shoshone Tribe, built free hot baths for men and women. They also built excellent camping facilities and community buildings to accommodate public functions for the locals and the seasonal influx of snowbirds, who arrived in October every year and generally stayed until April or early May.

This environment allowed Tecopa Hot Springs to do very well in spite of the continuing demise of Tecopa itself. With over 400 camper hookups, internationally recognized therapeutic hot mineral water, great climate, and cheap prices, Tecopa Hot Springs thrived. But in time, even the snowbirds faded away as a result of the collapse of services in Tecopa. This, and the refusal of the four business owners in Tecopa Hot Springs to upgrade services, created a freefall in the area's economy from which no return seemed possible.

By 1987, the lack of upkeep, poor maintenance of the hot baths, no repairs or replacement of structures, and a general malaise, led to the dissolution of the community's prior identity.

A new day had dawned for this historic community that, in truth, had so much to offer those willing to open their mind to its possibilities.

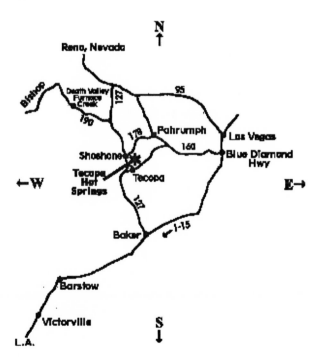

Chapter 3

Ruthie Badame

However rare true love may be, it is less so than friendship.
Francois DeLaRochefoucauld

Rumors traveled as fast as the local lizards. Everyone in Tecopa Hot Springs wanted to know why I had come and what I intended to do. Everyone could see things were rapidly changing. But in what direction, nobody knew.

I vaguely dreamed of a special place where people could come in feeling one way, and go away feeling a whole lot better with holistic treatment alone. I did have one small problem though; I had no firm idea of how to go about it, so I focused on first things first.

I began by picking up all the trash, and hauling it off so I could see just what I had. That kept us busy. Load after load made its way through Tecopa heading for the dump.

And people asked, "What's going on over there?"

And time after time I answered, "Just cleaning up the place."

One day as a group of people strolled by, a very sharply dressed, olive-skinned, feisty-looking lady with gray-streaked dark hair stepped out of the crowd. I guessed she was in her mid-seventies, though she certainly had a lot of energy. I had seen her before, and she had the look of a local leader. She had a very strong personality and radiated a kind of Eastern, city-type sophistication.

The day I first met Ruthie Badame, she wore a beautiful black and red outfit, topped off with a broad-brimmed hat. Although a bit out of place, I sensed this was not an unusual fashion statement for her, even in this rustic and remote locale. I loved her style.

From fifty feet away she yelled, "Hi!"

I don't know why but her brief greeting completely disarmed me and set me to smiling before I could even see her lovely Italian eyes. She continued to walk purposefully right up to me, extended her hand and asked, "Whatcha doin'?"

Sometimes you just know that you know. Ruthie and I both knew somehow that this would begin a friendship.

She said very simply, "I'm Ruth Badame. I live over there." She pointed to a small trailer at Delights Spa, just north of my facility. Up close I could see the Italian descent all over her face, and I detected an Eastern accent.

It turned out that many years ago, a friend of hers had traveled out West and found Tecopa Hot Springs, and the quality of the water and the desert location impressed her immensely. Knowing of Ruthie's worsening health, she suggested that Ruthie try Tecopa Hot Springs.

Ruthie, a successful businessperson in Philadelphia, Pennsylvania, took the advice of her friend and went to Tecopa for a visit and simply never left. She had healed. For her, the place was a miracle.

Once we shook hands she said, "You're Mr. Graham. They say you're an actor."

"Yes, I'm Cano Graham, but on the second point, well, I used to be a runner too, but I've decided that I'm not a runner if I'm not running, and I'm not an actor if I'm not acting! What is–is, and I *is* here." I smiled and shrugged my shoulders.

Her eyes sparkled.

"What are you building?"

39

"This is gonna be a Healing Center." I waved my arm to include all of my property.

"Oh?" She continued, encouraging me to explain further.

"Mrs. Badame, let me explain it this way…"

"First, please call me Ruthie," she interjected.

"Fine. Then please call me Cano."

"As I was saying, Ruthie, let me describe it by telling you a short story about an old Italian man who was a sculptor."

She smiled at my reference to the old Italian man. Ruthie was a great audience.

"One day this boy passed by an old Italian man who sat on top of a huge granite boulder, just chipping away. The boy yelled up, 'Whatcha making?' The old man cupped his hands and yelled back, 'I'm making an elephant!'"

"The boy responded, 'How're you gonna do that, mister?' The old man replied, 'I'm gonna chip away everything that doesn't look like an elephant!' And that, Ruthie, is how I'm going to build my Wellness Center. I'm just going to keep carving away everything that doesn't feel and act like a healing center."

She loved the little story, but I imagine she'd heard the parable before.

Then I offered, "Ruthie, how'd you like to seal our first meeting with a cup of coffee?"

That was the beginning of our friendship.

She soon became an enthusiastic supporter, and took it on herself to tell the whole world about the center for holistic medicine I was building. She became a one-woman public relations firm for all of my efforts.

Ruthie amazed me. She'd show up with a dozen or so tourists, answer their questions, show them what we planned to build next, and basically gave guided tours of the place. She genuinely enjoyed acting as our official hostess and diligently sought out foreign tourists from Germany, France, Canada, Mexico, and Japan, who had come just for a day. Because of her, they ended up staying a week. We started getting letters from all over the world. I called her my umbilical cord to the outside world.

Sometimes I got so wrapped up in things that I didn't take the time to eat. Then I'd look up and see Ruthie on her way with a plate of delicious homemade food. Only Ruthie could make me stop and eat.

Chapter 4

Sand Down A Rat Hole

Prosperity doth best discover vice; but adversity doth best discover virtue.   Sir Francis Bacon

I had been in Tecopa Hot Springs alone for a week, holed up in my little house on the corner. A long, hot summer lay ahead. Joyce was in Pasadena taking care of her active practice as a Yoga instructor. I missed her level-headedness because my head was anything but level. Everything was dead as yesterday's newspapers, and my brain was in the same condition.

The weather grew hotter the snowbirds had begun to leave, and I had the gut feeling that far more was wrong than I could see. I hadn't done a very good job of keeping track of the books, but nonetheless, the bucks just seemed to evaporate and I couldn't see much in the way of results. Nothing added up.

I was missing supplies, and my manger had no answers. I had stretched myself too thin between my mom, *the biz*, and dealing with all the issues at Tecopa Hot Springs. My mom would describe this type of situation as, "Pouring sand down a rat hole." That cliché also perfectly described my state of mind.

I had six cups of coffee and a fat roach or two, but nothing changed my mood. I only thought harder about what bothered me, but found no solution.

First I heard a horn honk, followed by a hard rap on the door and a loud, "Hi, Mr. Graham!"

I mumbled, "That's all I need, some company, especially some cheerful type." I didn't want anyone to know I was around! Oh, well, screw it, I'll shake 'em off quick, and get back to the occupation of being miserable. I had gotten very good at misery lately.

I opened the door and found a very busy lady, Ruthie Badame, rushing by me, singing out, "Hi, Cano. Lunchtime! You haven't stepped foot out of this door for the last twenty-four hours. What did I hear you call it just a few weeks ago, a severe sinking spell?"

I stepped out of the flow of traffic as she passed by me in the doorway, carrying an ice chest. I hadn't yet said a word, as I stood in awe. She continued, "What we have here is a particular meal that my father used to love on certain days. I think you're having one of 'em now. Did you even realize how nice it is outside today?" She finally glanced at me.

"Why yes, I ..."

She broke in, "Well, no matter. You've been cooped up in here, and I know that you don't cook too much so I thought to myself, 'I'll bet Cano would like some of this.' So here I am!"

I hadn't even had a chance to say, "Come in." I just sat there watching her unpack her ice chest of prepared food

She proceeded to get the dishes, glasses, and silverware out of my cupboard. In a twinkle, she had the table completely set, with everything in its proper place.

Before sitting down she said, "Would you mind if I leave the door open for awhile? It smells, well, funny in here."

She obviously referred to the lingering smell of the roaches I had smoked earlier.

I tried to make light of an embarrassing situation, "Sure, sure, no problem. That's a special natural herb I use on unique occasions. Nice fragrance, huh?"

She laughed. "I won't get a heroic case of the munchies just by breathing in here?"

"Ruthie, you know about the munchies?"

"Cano, you're so square at times. I may be 20 years older than you, but I probably knew about the munchies before you did. Just because I know about certain things doesn't mean that I practice them. I get the feeling that you try everything once."

I pretended resentment. "Now wait a second, Ruthie! That statement borders on being a bit harsh."

"A bit of hash or harsh?"

I busted out laughing, the first time I'd laughed in weeks, and it felt good.

She grinned, set a plate in front of me, and busily waved me off. "Never mind, never mind. Eat, my complex friend, eat and then I think it's time to talk."

"Talk? About what?" I didn't want to get into the conversation about what I'd just been thinking. Talking is bad for thinking. The process exposes all the flaws in the brain. I hadn't really isolated my thoughts. How can you identify shotgun pellets?

She didn't allow me any room to back off. "Want to talk now? Fine." Ruthie was on a roll. "Cano, at the café last night you mentioned that establishing communication with Las Vegas was essential.

"Yep. Nothing new there though. Just common sense. We need 'em."

She shrugged a shoulder, "No question about that point. I mean, it's obvious. But I've been thinking seriously about an issue that you need to address and as soon as possible."

"Oh really? What's up?"

She grew far more businesslike, and minced no words. "I feel your first real communication should start closer to home."

"What do you mean?"

"Bottom line: It's time for you to know a lot better just who's who in our town."

"Well I've met several. I mean I haven't gotten to know them very well I must admit, but I'm getting acquainted."

"Dear, as Art Babbit would say, 'You need to know who's *really* in your corner.'"

"Well, I must say."

"And Cano, others agree with me."

"Makes good sense! I'd appreciate it very much. But first, who are the others?"

"My best friends here, all my age or older, and they were here when I came. I believe you know them, or at least have seen them. First, there's Art and his wife, Luella, the Babbits."

"Yes, I met them. He's the ex-miner and boxer, and she's the schoolteacher? I believe they play bluegrass together, don't they?"

"Yep. They've been here a long time. Retired. Art thinks that you're going to be good for the community, but he doesn't trust your manager."

"I've got the same feeling."

"Then there's Sylvia Burton."

"She's one of my favorites! A lovely person."

Ruthie smiled. "She and Beulah Rosenberg are practically legends here. Sylvia is an artist and does quite well. Also she has a son about your age who's a highway patrolman. The way she carries herself is no accident. She used to be a well-known belly dancer."

"Sylvia? A belly dancer? Whoa, that's too much!"

For a few seconds I imagined how Sylvia must have looked sixty years ago, dancing in those rough clubs with her hips and long legs sliding all over the place.

"Cano, Cano, what are you thinking about?"

"Sylvia! The lady is something else!"

"And she can still dance too! She danced for several of us last year. She's such a delight!"

"How old is she?"

"She doesn't hide her age. She's 80 or 81."

"Unbelievable. Who are the others?"

45

"Well, two, Mori Rubenstein and Beulah Rosenberg."

"Little guy? Lotta energy? He's been over a few times to just talk. Talks about using clay to heal things. By the way have you heard about that? He even talks about drinking that stuff. He's got me curious."

"I understand. Yes, Mori's got a lot of energy and a lot of sense. I know a couple of the old-timers who swear by the clay, but I don't know much about it. Mori taught at a university in New York. He thinks you're going to get something done here. He's a health nut."

"I can tell. We need more like him." Then I joked, "Is he also clairvoyant and able to tell me what I'm going to do?"

Ruthie grew serious. "No he isn't. But he feels the way you're starting is correct. We all trust Mori. He's smart about things.

"Ruthie, you mentioned others. Who else? This Beulah, do I know her? I don't recall ever meeting her."

"You haven't yet. She's been in Long Beach for a few months, but she's heard about you. She's been here longer than anyone. Her husband was a superintendent, building the railroad from Death Valley through Tecopa to Barstow, hauling Borax. He drowned in a flash flood just outside of town. She's been the community leader for a long time, and we all feel that she's very important to what you want to do, whatever you decide to do."

I nodded. "I got it. How old is Beulah?"

"Beulah is 85. She uses a walker, but rest assured, she's sharp as a tack and nothing gets done without her say so. Mori said that she's curious about just what you're going to build."

"Aren't we all? All I can do is just keep chipping away."

Ruthie smiled. "Beulah doesn't know you yet, but the rest of us feel good about how you treat the older ones."

"Ruthie, I appreciate that, but how can I ask you all to help? I've been in kind of a rut myself lately."

" We're thinking that in a few weeks, after the season ends and the snowbirds leave, we'd like to get together and thoroughly

46

discuss what you'd like to do, to really understand what you have in mind. We'd like you to meet Beulah Rosenberg. She'll be back soon from Long Beach."

"Sounds great! " I was pleased to realize they had so much interest in me.

"Oh, I'm so glad you feel that way. Some thought you'd feel as if we were getting into your business."

"Oh no Ruthie, that's not it at all. Part of the whole problem for me is sensing that somehow the whole community can create together what can never be done individually. But I'm still sort of an outsider, you know? By the way, how do you see all of us getting together?"

"How about in two or three weeks for a Saturday or Sunday afternoon?"

"Sounds good. How about a Sunday afternoon dinner?"

Ruthie said, "Perfect. We'll need some time to really settle down and talk, to get acquainted, not just sit down and eat, then leave."

"Makes sense. Don't you all go to church?"

"Yes, we do. We could meet after church and discuss things over a late afternoon dinner."

I had an idea that involved my ace in the hole. "Ruthie, how does this sound? You've heard me talk about my mother quite a bit."

"Oh, yes. I wish we could meet her."

"Well that's just it. I could bring her up so you could all meet her. In fact she'd love to fix dinner for the group."

"We wouldn't want her to go through all that."

"You don't know her. She'd love it. She could fix fried chicken with all he trimmings. Tell you what, have someone fix dessert and a salad."

"Yes! Sylvia would love to do it! Cano, this is shaping up to be a fun Sunday with enough quality time to get well acquainted."

"Perfect. Two or three weeks gives us enough time so Mom

47

and everyone else can make plans. It also gives me enough time to, you know, focus on things."

After a few fruitful hours, she packed her ice chest and got ready to leave.

"Thanks so much for being you Ruthie. I feel much better. You came along at just the right time."

"Thank you, dear. We feel the same about you. We want Beulah to meet you. We'll keep our fingers crossed."

I grabbed her ice chest and walked her to the car. She was inside the car and had started the engine when she looked up at me. With those sparkling brown eyes reflecting her confidence, Ruthie said, "Keep chipping away, Cano."

"You're too much. " I bent over and kissed her cheek. "See ya later Ruthie."

"Bye, Cano."

I thought, "My God, this lady just rescued me."

Chapter 5

A Cross to Bear

Nothing is at last sacred but the integrity of your own mind.
Ralph Waldo Emerson

The phone rang as Ruthie left. I picked it up to hear the voice of Dick Collins, a Highway Patrolman, calling from Death Valley Junction. "Mr. Graham, this is Dick Collins with the Highway Patrol. I've got a tough situation here. A couple in their mid-thirties with three kids just lost their pickup, and most everything else in a fire at the Junction. They're on their way to Bakersfield, seems they came out from Missouri. I was getting ready to call the County to take 'em in and do something, but Art Babbit wanted me to call you."

"Well, I don't know what I might do, Dick. Could you put Art on the line and let me hear what he's got in mind?"

A husky voice said, "This is Art Babbit."

"Hi, Art, this is Cano. What's going on? I hear there's a problem."

"Yes, the situation is difficult. This here young family just lost everything they own when their old truck caught on fire. They're heading for Bakersfield. They weren't hurt in the fire, but I think that they've been on the road for quite a spell, and been camping out because they're a mess. They're just across the road from me.

"They had stopped for water when the fire started. The kids don't look well. I don't believe any of 'em have bathed in quite a spell. They all look scared and hungry, and smell sort of ... earthy."

I said, "Sounds as if someone's going to have their hands full."

"Cano, the man said he don't want no handouts. Says he wants to work. As I'm talking to you, he's standing there with his Bible in hand, lookin' like he's waitin' for a miracle of some kind. I wish you could see this deal, looks like something out of a Steinbeck story, *Tobacco Road* or the like."

"Damn, how old are the kids, Art?"

"Oh. I'd say the two little ones are six or seven, a boy and a girl. The older boy must be 13 or 14, and he sure needs a skin doctor. His face is sort of bad. He has infected pimples or something."

"Art, how much work does he want and for how long?"

"He just wants work so as to feed his family and get on to Bakersfield. He's dead set on getting to Bakersfield. Don't ask me why, guess it has to do with a job of sorts that's waiting for him."

"Well, I don't know. You know I had those big mine beams brought in to make a sign. Bill's busy starting on the new hot tub, and I sure don't want to break his rhythm or anything like that."

Art laughed. "Yeah, well that's some rhythm he's got going."

I asked, "Does he look like he's a boozer or doper?"

"Naw. I think that the best thing he could do is to take a stiff swig to clear his head, but no, he ain't no drinker. He looks more like a preacher that had his church burned down. Excuse me, Cano, I'm not making fun, it's just that this is some scene. I don't think they've eaten anything for a while. They've only made 75 miles in the past few days. Constant problems with the truck."

"Art, are you in your van?"

"Yes, Luella an' me was a comin' back from Independence."

"Art, I understand the situation. The fact is that I've got a

50

week's work and an old trailer for them to stay in. I'm sure we can figure a way to get 'em to Bakersfield when they get squared away, so no problem. Can you haul them down here? And what about their stuff?"

"There's not much left, just a suitcase or so. He tried to save the old truck and some of his things, but before he realized he couldn't do anything, hell, the whole thing went up. I've got plenty of room in the van. Be there in about 45 minutes or so."

I was sitting outside when Art and Luella rolled in with the family. When they all stepped out of the van the thought crossed my mind that this was more like *Grapes of Wrath* than *Tobacco Road*. Bless their hearts; they'd been to hell and back. I wondered what they'd experienced during the past few weeks, or months.

The man stood six feet, and weighed about 165 pounds or so, and had long, straight brown hair. The wife weighed in at about 120 pounds and stood about 5'8". She also had long straight brown hair. The older boy looked like his dad. The little ones just looked unconcerned, like everything was normal.

Art said, "Mr. Graham, this is the Hadley family. This here's Claude and his wife Helen. The boy is Hugh, and the young' 'uns are Misty and Greg."

"Hi, folks, sorry to hear that you've had such a bad break with the truck. First, Mr. Hadley, I do have some work for a few days, maybe a week or so, and would appreciate another hand. Mrs. Hadley, I just spoke with my manager's wife, and we have a trailer for your family to stay in, so that won't be a problem. Is that suitcase all you were able to save?"

Mrs. Hadley said, "Yes, sir, this is it. It's full of pictures and stuff."

"You lost all the clothes?"

"It all happened so fast. It was burnin' underneath, and all of a sudden it just went up in a blaze."

Art said, "It seems that there was some gasoline in the truck bed. It didn't take long. By the way, Claude's arm's burned. I didn't realize it until a few minutes ago. It needs attention."

"It looks like several things need attention. Do you think we should take him to Pahrump for the arm?"

Art said, "I don't think so. I'm going over to Sylvia's house and get some burn cream. Be right back."

Sylvia's house wasn't 125 yards away. Art and Luella returned, along with Sylvia, in a few minutes.

Art said, "Mrs. Hadley, this lady is a good friend of ours. She's here to help. Her name is Mrs. Burton."

Sylvia said, "Hi Cano," and then directed her attention to Claude's arm. "Could I see the burned place?"

Claude said, "Ma'am, I don't believe in doctors of no kind."

Sylvia quickly understood, and in a poised, thoughtful manner set the family at ease. "We all understand that, Mr. Hadley. What we have for a burn like that isn't medicine or a drug. It's just a type of natural healing earth. Nothing has been added. Some of us have used it for years to stop pain, and heal many things." She stepped a few feet to the van, and came out with a big bowl of her burn cream. At that time I didn't realize what she had in the bowl, I just watched the moment unfold.

Claude said, "What's in that stuff, Ma'am?"

"A type of clay."

"Clay? You mean clay like Jesus put in the blind man's eyes?"

Sylvia glanced at me, then at Art and Luella, and back to Claude. "Yes, I suppose it's very similar, when I think about it."

I turned a bit and whispered to Art, "Is that the stuff you've all been talking about?"

"That's it."

"And the stuff works on burns?"

Art nodded. "Yes. Have you seen his arm? He's burned pretty good, and not a peep out of him. C'mon, let me show you this."

I stood fascinated, "Claude, could I see your arm?

"Yes, sir. Here it is." The man was burned badly on the right hand and forearm. Sylvia waited patiently for him to answer either yes or no.

Mrs. Hadley came over to Sylvia, Art, Luella, and me while we stood examining the arm, and said, "Claude, me an' the kids been prayin' on it, and we believe you should do this."

Claude said, "Me too. It ain't like it's from a doctor, or a drugstore or such. I mean, after all, it's in the Bible. And, Helen, have you noticed something? This place sort of looks like what I always figured the place where Jesus was from looked like. I mean the desert and all."

Art, Luella, Sylvia, and I just looked at each other and waited for the moment to play out.

Claude walked over to us and said, "Mrs. Burton, I'd mightily appreciate it if you'd allow me to use that there burn cream. Would you do it for me? Just whatever it is you do. It's startin' to hurt more."

This was better than any movie scene I'd ever witnessed. I was watching high drama. I turned my head and quietly said, "Art, you're not concerned with infection?"

He said, "Cano, just hold on. Mori, Sylvia, Luella, and me have been using this stuff for years and have found the opposite. This has soaked up and stopped any infection we've ever seen. We don't know how, but it damn sure does it. Watch. I've seen Sylvia work before."

Sylvia held the trembling arm with her left hand while Helen and the kids stood close by for moral support. We all knew that he was in absolutely excruciating pain, but he endured without a whimper, but I saw the clenched muscles in his jaw. In a calm and gentle voice Sylvia said, "Mrs. Hadley, you might want to tell the children that this holy substance will quickly make their father feel better."

Then she dipped her hand into the bowl of gelled clay, drew out a big handful, and with one confident stroke back and forth, covered the man's hand and forearm.

As fast as a man would react to thrusting his hand into a bucket of ice water, he drew back in astonishment, and began repeating, "Praise God, Praise God, Praise God."

The scene of Claude burying his head in Sylvia's shoulder, repeating his prayer, with Helen, Mark, Misty and Greg surrounding and holding them both, is forever burned into my memory.

I cleared my throat and swallowed. "Damn! Whew! I'm glad I saw that in person."

Art said, "That's what we're talking about, Cano."

Little did I know how that scene would affect my life. My priorities immediately shifted.

Sylvia called a few hours later, and said that while getting the children and Helen cleaned up, she gave Helen and Mark a facial. During that process, she realized that Mrs. Hadley had a bad yeast infection.

I asked, "What should be done? I don't know anything about such things."

Sylvia said, "It's a female infection, though Claude is probably infected as well. I know from friends that the clay will take care of it. I think they're already feeling better." Before the Hadley's went to bed that night, Luella Babbit made some calls. After a personal visit to a few families in Tecopa, she returned with adequate clothes for the whole family. Not an extravagant display, but enough. Not thrown in a box, but ironed and on hangers. And, after soaking Claude's arm and reapplying the clay, he enjoyed some pain-free rest.

The next morning, Mori called. "Mr. Graham, I understand you saw our clay in action yesterday?"

I said, "Well, yes I did. It worked on a burn, and I don't think burns like that are so easy to treat. The stuff stopped the pain. That alone is remarkable. Will it really help to heal the arm?"

Mori said, "You won't believe it until you see the results. Interesting isn't it?"

I said, "Yes, it is. What's in that stuff? Surely all clay won't do that?"

"Obviously not."

I said, "By the way, Sylvia said the lady had a yeast infection, and from what she said, I guess it was no problem to clear it up with the clay."

"Yep, the women hereabouts have used the clay for feminine hygiene for years."

"Well, I'll be. That's interesting!" I laughed. "I'm beginning to see why you guys live so long around here."

"You'd be surprised how many 'round here don't know about the stuff, or just don't care. It's just here. Snowbirds pick it up by the sack full, and take it home with 'em."

"Well, I guess every area has a folk medicine of some kind that a few swear by."

He grimaced at my description of folk medicine. "Mr. Graham, several of us feel that the importance of this deposit of clay is far more significant than to describe it as folk Medicine."

"Sorry. I don't mean to treat the subject lightly, but has it ever been tested clinically? I mean, there's a great need for things that heal people."

"Mr. Graham, that's exactly what we're trying to interest you in. You've said you want to build a healing center. Well, a few of us know that this is a healing substance. Hell, the local Indians have known it for years. And, I might add, a few of us have used it on several different types of problems."

"Well Mori, I certainly do appreciate all of you bringing this to my attention. The subject deserves some serious consideration. I don't know if we could use the stuff in a modern therapeutic setting, but it's sure something to look into."

"Well, if you have any questions about anything, please call me. Oh yes, I meant to add, many of us have used it quite successfully for dental problems, and through doing that we have found that it's very effective for stomach problems. Anyway, I'm glad you got to see it work. I enjoy talking to you about the stuff. "By the way Cano, did you have any problem at your place last night?"

"No, why?"

"Some drunks tore down our little cross on the hill last night. It was old and leaning, but at least it was there. Well, it's history now. Just a little cross, made of two by fours, it wasn't very strong, but we all liked our little cross up on the hill. These young punks from Las Vegas come out, use our hot baths, get drunk, then tear down our cross!"

I said, "Well Mori, some just like to destroy things."

He said, "Yes, I know, but our cross wasn't a religious cross. They put 'em on hills around here to indicate the presence of water. It's a marker for water. It started way back in the early days to guide miners to water. Anyway, it's down."

"That's a shame. It looked good up there."

"Well, anyway, you got to see what me, Art, and Sylvia have been talking about. G'bye."

"Goodbye, Mori, and thanks again."

I found myself thinking, I wish he hadn't included all the other uses. Who in Hell would believe all this? It's just too much. I needed to do some serious thinking about whether to stay or not, and he's talking about a primitive cure-all. Jesus! What next?

The next morning I had the workers together that I'd hired to build a big sign out of mine beams. I had a great idea for a sign. I was going over my drawing of the sign, when down the road came Claude.

"Hi Claude! How's the arm?"

He smiled like a young opossum eating green persimmons. "Mr. Cano, this here ain't no problem. The Lord provides. Yes, sir, the Lord provides. I'm ready to work. What are ya'll a'buildin'?"

"It's gonna be a nice big sign. Right here on the corner, out of those mine beams."

Claude said, "Whoa, that'll be a heck of a sign. What can I

do?"

"It'll be an hour or so before we start. You guys just sort of hang loose and have a cup of coffee."

Chuck, a thoughtful man who had found a home in the desert, walked over to Claude and said, "Hi Claude, I'm Chuck. I heard about what your family went through, and I'm sure sorry. I hear you're going to Bakersfield before too long?"

"That's the plan. It's been quite a journey, but we're almost there."

Chuck said, "It so happens that I'm going to Tehachapi next week, and Bakersfield's just over the mountain from there, so your family is more than welcome to ride along."

"My goodness! The Lord does provide! Thanks so much. Bless you!" Claude was so grateful.

Chuck said, "Sorry to hear you lost your truck and everything in the fire, bad break."

We all stood within earshot when Claude said, "Oh thanks, Chuck. But these folks have been real good to us. It's just a cross I have to bear. We'll make it."

I turned to the workers and asked, "What'd he say?"

Chuck turned to me and asked, "Who?"

"Claude. What'd he say about the cross?"

Chuck replied, "Oh, he mentioned a cross he had to bear."

"A cross?" I asked. I wheeled, went into the house, and started drawing. A few minutes later, I poked my head out of the door and said, "Hey Chuck! Have we got everything ready to go for the sign?"

"Yes. Bolts, saw, posthole digger, cement, all ready to go."

"Have we got any white paint in the tool shed?"

"Yeah, but I thought you were going to leave it natural!"

"I've changed my plan. We're going to build us a nice, pretty white cross."

"A cross? Where?"

I pointed up on the hill, "Up there where the old one stood, except when we get through, no one will ever tear it down again. They'd have to dismantle half the hill!"

"How's that?"

"Because we're going to build this one out of mine beams and railroad timbers, all bolted and braced together, and anchored in the big rocks, with a couple hundred pounds of cement!"

Everyone yelled at once, "Yeah! Yeah! Yeah!"

It didn't take long to cut the timbers to fit snug, drill holes for the bolts, and get the five-gallon buckets ready to carry the cement up the hill. Seven men carried the assembled cross up the hill, on their backs and shoulders. I took a picture of the scene. Claude positioned himself in the middle of the front three going up the hill. Halfway up, they set it down to rest. By this time, a good-sized crowd had gathered to watch and the men waved to friends and spectators below.

Then Claude yelled down in a strong voice, "Hey, Mr. Graham! It ain't hard to bear this cross."

With that the workers waved proudly and proceeded the rest of the way up the hill to set our community's new cross in place.

Mori, Sylvia, Luella, and Art had watched the entire scene and walked up behind me.

Art said, "Cano, it's sure funny how some things turn out, ain't it?"

I turned around to face my friends. They all bore wide smiles that mirrored my own.

Chapter 6

My Ace In The Hole

All sorrows can be borne if you put them in a story or tell a story about them."
Isak Dinesen

The one great advantage I enjoyed in my life was having Eva Graham for a mother and knowing that she always understood, loved, and demonstrated her pride in me. On the surface, this may sound unwarranted, even unrelated to the subject of clay therapy, but rest assured that whenever you use clay to heal yourself, someone you love, or a stranger, remember you have this English/Welsh/Pennsylvania Dutch/Choctaw Indian woman named Eva Graham to thank. If you could have only met her, then you would know. She possessed a rare love for life, be it plant, animal, or person.

Eva Graham knew she was alive, and that this was her time. She was indeed, by any standard, a loving, vibrant, considerate, consistent, bright, and secure person, that dearly loved to *do* things. She loved to dance, and fish. She could do one all day and the other all night.

When I made my request for a dinner for my friends, she reacted exactly the way I thought she would. She grew excited as the prospect of coming to Tecopa Hot Springs and meeting my friends. Mother knew I wasn't happy overall with the way things were going in Tecopa, but rather than giving her specifics, I pretty much kept my opinion of the situation to the vague. "I'm just not sure that this is a reasonable investment."

Well aware of my interest in owning a spa of some type, as we had often discussed the idea, she also knew I had an acting career that deserved attention.

She looked forward to the trip as an adventure of sorts. She always traveled with a map to know where she was, and what lay ahead.

Mother never cared a great deal about the desert. She loved trees, flowers, and lots of green. In the beginning, the barren landscape intimidated her. She simply didn't feel the kindred spirit with the desert that she enjoyed elsewhere, but all that soon changed.

Mother had a great way of cutting to the truth of a situation, and I was curious about how she would critique what I was trying to create. I needed every advantage I could get. I wanted the leaders in Tecopa Hot Springs to get to know her, my Ace in the Hole.

Eighty-Five and Alive

And so we started on our journey to Tecopa Hot Springs on a Sunday morning. On the way, I suggested that we stop at the Green Tree Inn in Victorville, California for breakfast, her favorite meal of the day. What a great choice!

I recall how lovely she looked when we entered the restaurant. The aromas in the Green Tree were a mixture of good things that seems to exist in a facility that has a special quality to its food. As we entered the restaurant, mother turned her nose up in the air as if she were a mother wolf with her pup, testing the air for fresh game. She instantly nodded a positive response. The place on that Sunday morning had a large number of senior customers, three of whom were older gentlemen, handsomely dressed in western outfits.

Mother had just finished her sensory examination of the room, when one impressive fellow said, "Ma'am, don't matter how good it smells in here, it ain't any better than you looked getting' outta that pretty car!"

Now the reader must understand that Eva Graham loved cowboys, in fact, anything western. She'd read every book that Louis Lamour had ever written, and was the only person I knew who openly wept when John Wayne died.

This man was a big, good-looking 75-year old guy that wore his western clothes in a style that indicated he was no drugstore cowboy. Two other men at their large table joined in the appraisal and approval of my mother's virtues.

She loved it and smiled. "Thanks. I'll tell you fellows this much, this table is plumb full of good-looking cowboys, too."

With that several tables around the area started to applaud, and the three scooted over and asked us to join them for breakfast. Everyone had a delightful time. She was 85 and fully alive.

"Little Eva" in Action

When we left Victorville, I adjusted the radio to a station that featured oldies but goodies. She loved music, and we settled in for the rest of the three-hour trip.

Mother didn't like to go fast in a car because it frightened her. When traveling alone I moved along pretty well, but with her beside me, the habit of staying in the right-hand lane, and holding a steady 55 miles per hour always brought the response that I loved to hear: "Honey, you're such a good driver."

Ah, what I'd give to hear those words just one more time.

I began to think back, way back in time, then broke into my memories to ask, "Honey, do you remember when you stuck me with a safety pin?"

She laughed. "Oh Lord, you couldn't recall that. You were too young, just a baby."

"Baby or not, even then I knew it was an accident, but it still stung! And I remember when we went to the tomato patch, just you and me, and we came upon a rattlesnake!"

She turned the radio down and said, "You remember me killing the rattler?"

"Yes I do! You moved me back down the path and you went at him with the hoe. I remember it like it happened yesterday. You were in a frenzy!"

She puzzled. "You weren't but, well, let's see ... I was 34 or 35, so you couldn't have been more than four or five years old! You remember that?"

"Sure I do, but even before that rattlesnake I remember you canning some tomatoes. Seems to me like it took you a week!"

She looked as though she were folding back the pages of her life. "My, that was a long time ago. I canned twelve hundred jars."

I said, "You know mom, I'll never forget the sight of all those jars with tomatoes. And of going to bed with the sound of the pressure cooker screaming as if it were about to blow the house apart. The smell of tomatoes hung in the house like a liquid, tangy smoke."

"Honey, you weren't but about three or four years old!"

"It doesn't matter. I'd go to bed and you'd be watching that pressure cooker about to blow up, and jars everywhere. That smell will always be red to me. Then I'd wake up in the morning, and do you remember the sound of the mourning dove? And the oil well pumping up north? Anyway, I went downstairs, and there you were, still on your feet! I knew that you hadn't been to bed."

"I had to get 'em canned. They were ripe."

"Oh, I kind of knew that you had a lot to get done, but I never did understand the clothespins on your ears."

Mom laughed. "Dear Lord, I do remember that!"

I laughed too. "So do I, and when I asked about the clothespins on your ears you said, 'So I'll stay awake.' But you know, I really didn't understand until I went to the washstand, got a clothespin, and put it on my ear! It didn't hurt too much at first, but soon enough I was running around in pain trying to see how much I could take!"

By now mother was in stitches laughing at my description of the incident. Oh, how she loved to laugh!

"Do you remember when you cut your leg open on the paint can?"

I thought for a moment and said, "I sure do. You know what I remember? The cut didn't hurt nearly as bad as it looked, but it was the first time I saw you scared."

Mom said, "Oh yes, I was scared. We couldn't stop the bleeding. I was real scared. I was also scared when Frank burned himself on the stove. Do you remember that?"

"No I don't, but I do recall the time he drank some kerosene."

She shook her head. "What a time we had getting the cow milked so we could get some milk into him!"

When mom mentioned my brother getting burned, it made me think of Claude Hadley and his burn. I wondered how he was, and if that clay stuff had worked to help heal his arm. "Mom, have you ever heard of using clay to heal things?"

"Clay? Like plain clay? To heal? No, I can't say I have." Then she tossed her head back, laughed and said, "But I've eaten it before."

"You have? Why?"

"When I was carrying you, I kept a pan of black dirt and red clay under our bed. I had a strong craving for it. It smelled good, and I ate it!"

"Are you serious? You ate dirt and red clay when you carried me?" Then I joked, "What have you done to me? Well, I'll be. You never told me about that before."

She shrugged. "I just never thought about it."

"Where'd you get it?"

"Where? Honey, it was everywhere! Daddy brought me some good black dirt, and the red clay was all around."

"Why sure, there was a lot of reddish-orange ground all around our place, and on the roads."

She loved this memory, "Yep, that was red clay. I hated it in my garden, but I loved it when I carried you!"

"That's wild! You eating clay."

"Oh, it's not that unusual, many women do it when they're pregnant. I've known about that for a long time. Women all over the world do it. I once read about that subject in one of your father's *National Geographics*."

"How much farther to go?"

"Not too much farther, just over those hills. You know Mom, that's sort of a coincidence."

"What is?"

"Well, you eating clay when you were carrying me, and now I find that they eat clay up here, and use it to heal wounds and things. Man, I think that borders on being a little bit strange."

"Your friends up here use clay to heal wounds. What kind of clay? Is it red clay?"

"No, sort of grayish-green. They say it works on lots of things. They even put it on burns."

She checked her map to see where we were. "This desert is kind of nice. Different isn't it? I think we're getting pretty close."

I liked watching her study the road map. I imagined her as a young girl studying maps of far away places, and dreaming unspoken dreams of adventure. She contented herself by finding adventure and worth in each new day wherever she was.

"Yes honey, you're right, we're close now." We were headed North on Highway 127, about 10 miles south of Tecopa. I had prepared mother for what she'd see when we crested the hill, and dropped down into the huge, ancient lakebed surrounded by mountains on all sides except on the North. This was home to Tecopa Hot Springs, and Tecopa and Shoshone, California.

"See there, honey? About halfway up those hills? That's where the waterline was for the old lake. See it?"

"Yes, I think I do. My goodness, your father would have loved this! This must have been a very large lake. How far north did it go?"

"I'm not sure. I think about forty miles or so. When we get close to Tecopa, you can look south, and clearly see where thousands of years ago the washout occurred, and the cliffs gave way causing the whole lake to drain. Must have been a sight!"

"This is something! This is where you want to build a healing center? Oh, I like it! There's something about this area."

Oh how I loved sharing my life and dreams with her.

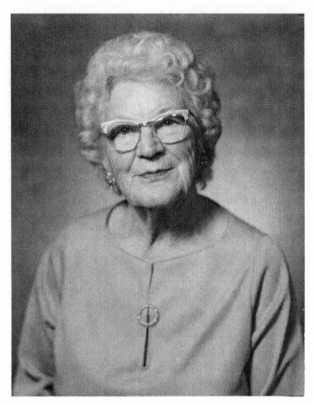

Eva Graham (1902 – 1992)

About Eva Graham

I sometimes wonder:
Who would I be,
or want to do,
or care to give
if not what
she believed I was?

Cano

Chapter 7

Coincidence: How Things Just Seem to Happen.

Our destiny rules over us even when we are not yet aware of it; it is the future that makes laws for us today.

Friedrich Wilhelm Nietzsche

Ruth Badame and Sylvia Burton pulled into the parking area before I got the car unpacked. Mother was already inside going through drawers and cupboards to see what she had to work with.

Ruthie, Sylvia, and I went inside. "Mom, I want you to meet two friends of mine."

They loved Mom as soon as they saw her. She always projected an attitude that said she wanted to know you.

"Sylvia Burton, Ruthie Badame, this is my mom, Eva Graham."

Sylvia said, "Eva, its so good to meet you. Cano has told us a lot about you, and we've grown fond of your son. That makes it all the more important to welcome you to Tecopa Hot Springs."

Mom said, "Well, thank you. He's told me about you folks too. It doesn't surprise me to meet you two first. You're the first ones he told me about. Will the others be along before too long?"

Ruthie answered, "Yes Eva, it won't be but a few minutes before Art and Luella Babbitt arrive. I just talked to them, and Mori Rubenstein should be picking up Beulah Rosenberg any time now. They'll be along soon. What can we do to help?"

Mom said, "Oh, there's not that much to do. What time do you think everyone would like to eat and how many will we have for dinner?" She wanted to know exactly what she was dealing with before she relaxed. Ruthie said, "Oh, I think later on in the afternoon will be fine, and I think we'll have eight. Cano says you're fixing chicken?"

Mom said, "Just plain old chicken. I'm so glad that we can eat later on. That gives me a chance for a good visit."

Sylvia said, "Yes it does, and don't worry about dessert Eva. I've baked a special cake. I think you'll like it. I'll go across the road later on and get it."

Ruthie jumped in and said, "And I've got a salad all ready to mix up, so don't worry about that either."

Mother said, "Well, isn't that nice."

A sudden knock on the door demanded our attention.

Ruthie said, "That's Art and Luella. I can tell their knock anywhere. It's as if he's trying to break down the door."

Sylvia, closest to the door, opened it for the newcomers. I had already mentioned to mom about Art and Luella's music, so Art and mother hit it off immediately. I knew they would.

Art, hefty around the waist, had a full beard, and wore one of those wide leather belts. Luella was small and quiet. Both were attractive in their own way, but if you met them separately you'd never imagine these two as a couple until you listened to them discuss something.

These two were doers. Art was very familiar with Indian culture, having lived on a Reservation during his early years. Luella was a retired schoolteacher, and as soft spoken as Art was robust. She and Art were always ready to play a little bluegrass. They could bring the house down when Luella got busy keeping time with an old tambourine banging against her hips while Art knocked out a tune with his fiddle.

Art couldn't wait. "Eva, Cano tells me that he's got some Choctaw Indian blood from you."

Mom saw it coming. "Yes, sir, we sure are proud of it!"

"Good to hear, I'm Cherokee."

Mom didn't know just where this was going. "You know, I've never heard a Cherokee play the fiddle."

"Well, Eva, you're a gettin' ready to."

With that Art went to their van, and in a matter of a few minutes, mother and Sylvia were up and dancing to Art's fiddle, with Luella's tambourine flying off her hips. The joint was jumping. The best times are never planned, they just happen. We were all taking a break when Mori and Beulah arrived.

The scene unfolded as if a large, female, four-star general, entered a battlefield command post, tugging her small driver alongside. I fully expected someone to bark, "Atten-shun!" and command everyone to snap to until the follow-up "At-ease." For a split second, Beulah inspected her troops while Mori assisted Beulah with her walker.

In another split second Beulah relaxed and said, "Hi everyone, we got here just as soon as we could."

In those few seconds, Beulah Rosenberg established herself as the matriarch she had been for the last fifty years. Mori Rubenstein, very much of a take-charge kind of guy, had a feisty air about him that some small wiry guys have. One minute in any crowd and everybody knew him as a sharp, highly educated person, given to testiness.

Ruthie said, "I've got something that will go good with coffee." And out of a straw basket she took some freshly baked oatmeal cookies.

We all looked forward to the next few hours. Conversation came easy, and didn't flow in any particular direction. Everyone was just getting to know each other. Beulah and I sensed we had to match up sooner or later.

Art changed the momentum when he asked, "How's it going for you Cano? Have you decided on the number of rentals you're going to build?"

He had pinned me quick. I wasn't ready to answer the question. I had far too much on my mind.

"No, I haven't. I'm in the process of building a hot tub right now, and I kind of want to see how that goes before I jump into putting a new roof over the swimming pool, and bringing in more rental units."

Mori asked, "A new roof over your pool? That'll be real nice, but who's going to do it?"

Art said, "That'll be a job. Anyone in mind?"

"No. Not yet. I need someone to oversee the work. I'm not too comfortable with Bill. He doesn't seem to take to that kind of work. I've also got some other interests in Los Angeles that I'd like to tend to, so I can't be looking over his shoulder every day."

Art said, "So, you're lookin' for somebody that can git done what you wanna' git done."

"That's about the size of it."

Art looked at Sylvia and then back at Mori, back to Ruthie, and then to Beulah while Luella watched me.

I saw a silent vote taken, and a look in the eye of each dictated the verdict.

Beulah said, "Mrs. Graham, I suppose you're wondering why we're so interested in what your son is doing, even though we don't know yet just exactly what it is."

"Well, it seems to me that as long as you folks have been here, you have a right to know anything that you want to know, whenever you want to know it." Mom fired straight from the hip, and they loved it. Mori said, "So really you're just kind of trying to figure out what type of service you're going to offer?"

"That's about it, Mori. When I get some of the basics finished, the hot tub and swimming pool, then I'll decide on some therapeutic service that isn't offered in the area now. Maybe a clinic for various types of holistic medicine. I'm undecided, but by the end of the summer, I'll know in what direction I want to go."

Beulah fired the first shot at me. "Cano, you haven't been here through you're first summer yet, have you?" Her remark smacked of being close to a kind of threat, or promise of some kind. "We've seen several come and go. The first summer usually gets them."

All five sets of eyes studied me. They had just thrown down the gauntlet.

"If I fail, it won't be because of the temperature. I love this climate! There's different kinds of heat. Some bother me. Some don't." I was thinking of the legal kind. They were thinking about thermometers.

Art said, "Well, it looks to me that if you want to get something done with the pool and all, you're going to need a good, honest, hard-working man that ain't afraid of a little heat!"

Everyone in the room except mom and I already knew the answer. "There's a fellow who lives over in Pahrump that does a lot of work around here. His mom lives across the street there, around the corner from Sylvia. He's the best there is, and fair to boot. His name is Curt Hibdon, and he can do it all."

"I'm sure glad to know that there's someone local that you all think so highly of. I'd like to get in touch with him."

Art said, "I can fix that up in a few days."

"Thanks a lot!"

Beulah said, "Listen. I wanted to ask you all, who put the big cross up on the hill?"

Art replied, "Well, I guess that you could rightly say that Cano did that. Ain't it pretty?"

Beulah said, "It's beautiful. I've been trying to get A.V.R.A. to do that for a while, but we just couldn't seem to find the time or the energy. Thanks so much, Cano! What did you make it out of? Sure looks big and sturdy."

"It's made of old mine beams, and some of those railroad timbers from the wash north of town."

Beulah said, "Well, I'll say." She looked at everyone, "Can you imagine that? My husband was the foreman on the day that trestle was built. They hauled all of those timbers from Barstow.

He'd get a big kick out of you all doing that."

I said, "We had a family working here for a week or so, the Hadley's, and he said something that gave me the idea to do it. It was kind of like a happening of sorts. I was gonna build a sign, but it turned out to be a cross."

Mom said, "You didn't tell me about the cross."

"Well, it just kind of slipped my mind." I smiled. "Besides that, I'd rather show it to you than tell you about it anyway."

Beulah wanted to see the cross again from this side of the hill, so we all filed out the door to get a better view. Some of the local kids had put some strips of aluminum foil on the cross and a slight breeze caused reflections to ripple across it.

Mother said, "My Lord, it looks just like crystals hanging off it. Like a crystal cross!"

I suppose it's safe to say that our future name was created at that moment.

When we settled back down inside, mother started fussing in the kitchen, getting things ready to start frying the chicken, Mori said, "Cano, have you heard about A.V.R.A.?"

"I think Ruthie mentioned it, some local organization, like a civic club?"

Mori said, "In some sense I suppose, but it's more than that here. It's all we've got."

"If you're looking for a new member, I'm your man. I'd like to be a part of it."

Everyone was interested in what Beulah had to say, though she remained reticent. It was as if she had consciously decided to reserve her opinion for a while about A.V.R.A and me.

At the time, I didn't realize the importance of having A.V.R.A behind me. To have them leading the way like a Chamber of Commerce could mean so much, no matter what I decided to do. Later I realized A.V.R.A. was created to promote the area. This was exactly what my project needed, and my project was exactly what the community needed.

Art said, "Smells good, Eva!" Something about the aroma of mom's fried chicken got everyone's juices flowing. Cooking was an act of friendship for mother. She enjoyed the communion of preparing a meal for others.

As Luella and Sylvia set the table and got other dishes ready, Mori yelled across the room, "Eva, have you ever heard of using clay to heal things?"

Sylvia looked at mom, obviously waiting for an answer.

"No I haven't. Cano asked me the same question. I never used it to heal things but I've eaten it before! In fact, when I was carrying Cano, I ate a lot of it, red clay. I used to keep it under my bed in a pan. It satisfied my craving."

Art asked, "Where you folks from? Where was this red clay?"

Mom said, "Oklahoma-North Central grasslands. Lots of red clay there. Too much. Cano was born on a farm full of red clay."

Beulah said, "Eva, I'm from Oklahoma."

Art said, "Beulah, I thought that you moved out here from Barstow? Didn't you tell us that?"

"I did, but first I lived in Oklahoma, in a little town called Sand Springs."

Mother jumped in. "Sand Springs? Well for Lords sake! I grew up in Tulsa. Sand Springs sits just down the road!"

Beulah got caught up in the moment. "Well, can you just believe that? What a small world. I'll say!"

"Beulah, I think we're close to the same age. I'm eighty-five."

"I'm eighty-five, too! I went to school in Sand Springs."

Mom said, "I quit school early and went to work."

Beulah nodded. "A lot of us did. Eva, do you remember the flu epidemic in 1918?"

"You bet your life I remember! They hauled off people in wagons!"

"They sure did. I tell people that and they think I'm stretching the story!"

"Beulah, I can't get over this. Well I'll be! Isn't this

something?"

Beulah probed, "How old were you when you went to work?"

By this time everyone was captivated by their conversation.

Mom turned her chicken and some oil popped out of the skillet and burned her arm. She did what she always did when hot grease hit her arm. She gritted her teeth and half yelled, "SHHHIITT!!" Then just as quickly she faced the group and said, "I'm sorry, I forgot where I was. Sorry Beulah. Let's see. I was fifteen, just turned fifteen."

Beulah laughed. "I went to work when I was fourteen!"

Mother countered, "Well, the fact is that I was fourteen, and lied about my age so I could go to work for the phone company in Tulsa."

Beulah covered her mouth in shock. "No! You didn't!"

Flabbergasted, Mom asked, "Did you?"

"I sure enough did!"

Mom gasped. "You mean we worked at the phone company at the same time?"

Beulah said, "Well, it seems like it!"

"I don't remember you."

"I can't place you either."

Mom said, "I worked on long distance."

"I worked on local calls. Eva, do you remember the supervisor's name, the real large man?"

"Gibson! Fat Gibson!"

Beulah threw her arms in the air. "That's it! Fat Gibson! I'd forgotten!"

Mom turned to me and asked, "Have you got that picture of me when I was nineteen years old?"

"Sure do. It's in the bedroom, wait just a second."

I returned with my favorite picture of mom and handed it to Beulah.

She took one look and said, "That's little Evelyn! My God, Eva, you're little Evelyn! I remember you. You used to dance around all the time! You got in trouble with Fat Gibson for dancing one time!"

I thought mother would faint. "For God's sake, this is unbelievable!"

Everyone started clapping and laughing. "Beulah? Beulah? Did we call you Bea? Big Bea?"

"Yes! Everyone did. I'm Big Bea!"

By this time mother and Beulah had fallen into each other's arms while everyone else laughed, cried, yelled, and clapped.

"Unbelievable!"

"Can you imagine?"

"Evelyn, I just can't believe this! Am I dreaming? Has it been 70 years?"

"This is the strangest thing I've ever heard of. After all these years, to meet in the desert!" Mom hugged her and said, "Big Bea! I can't get over this. It's a...what do they call it when a strange thing happens? You know! Oh! What is it when things come together that aren't suppose to?"

Then Mori said, "I'll tell you this much, this day will forever change the way that I think about coincidence. I'm not so sure there is such a thing."

"Hell, me neither!" Art said, then he started fiddling, and Luella started banging on her hips with that old tambourine.

Good times aren't planned. They just happen. Just a coincidence? My Ace in the Hole was surely the wind beneath my wings, and she carries me even today.

I soon submerged myself in the discipline of using clay therapeutically. Healing with clay and building an alternative medical community became my passion. The following year, the fine people of Tecopa Hot Springs elected me president of A.V.R.A., which was Mori's idea all along. The community of Tecopa Hot Springs enjoyed a much-deserved prosperity.

Chapter 8

The Inventor

In things pertaining to enthusiasm, no man is sane who does not know how to be insane on proper occasions.

Henry Ward Beecher

"Mr. Graham, don't get me wrong, the clay you gave me a couple of weeks ago to try on my feet has worked wonders, for sure, and we truly appreciate your interest. No question. I can't believe the difference it's made in my feet in such a short time, it's amazing! But to suggest that my wife put the stuff on her abscessed tooth, well frankly, I think that's a bit too much. I mean, we're talking about clay."

Mrs. Simmons walked by us on the patio, getting our attention with her clay-covered face. Still new to me, the clay remained more of a novelty than a serious issue.

She waved and said, "Hi, guys."

Curious, I asked, "Where'd you get the clay?"

She kept walking. "Your maid gave me some."

I owed the man an explanation. "Mr. Simmons, I certainly understand what you're saying, and feeling. I mean, if I hadn't seen the stuff work myself on some things, and heard about its use for years around here for dental problems, well I'd have never recommended something that might have caused the slightest harm."

"Please...Cano, isn't it?"

"Yes, call me Cano. It's hard to remember, but it's my name. It's pronounced Cah-no. Okay?"

"Great, call me Al. All right, Cano, I'm glad you understand. I should explain. My main concern stems from Joan's allergies. We've spent a ton of money over the years trying to isolate and solve the problem. Doctors claim it's a combination of circumstances. To tell you the truth, I'm afraid she might be allergic to something in the stuff." His point struck me between the eyes. I got the point and felt foolish. "Well sure. I've obviously let my enthusiasm get ahead of me. Sorry."

I felt some relief about the whole subject. Partial relief, but certainly not total. By Al pulling me up on this matter, he rightly uncovered my serious need for a lot of sophisticated hard data about this stuff. I was going off like a kid playing Doctor, and now realized I had to get real.

Al tried to sooth my feelings. "Now understand, Cano, I'd bet a dollar to a dime that it wouldn't cause a problem, might even help. But I just can't take such a gamble. You understand." I said, "I'll tell you what. The next time you and your wife come out here, I'll have some answers if they exist, one way or another about the stuff." I shook my head in disbelief. "It's time for me to fish or cut bait on this deal! You know, Al, the more I think about it, the more ridiculous the whole subject becomes! Hell, I wouldn't dream of putting anything in my mouth without knowing what was in it."

I suddenly realized that this makeshift folklore medicine, the Clay, was full-time nonsense until I got some straight up answers.

Al tried to do his best. "Now, Cano, don't be too rough on yourself. No matter what you find out about the stuff, the stuff works! I've spent hundreds, if not thousands of dollars in the past ten or so years trying to get some relief for my feet. I hurt 'em when I was younger by wearing boots that didn't fit and working and standing on a cold concrete floor. About crippled me. Now, they're always sore, and getting worse. It sort of scares me. I'm still standing a lot at work, but at least it's on carpet. I work at the Tropicana, and so does Joan. Anyway, my foot doctor says that it's arthritis now. We've been coming here for the past six or seven years, long before you bought the place and this hot mineral water has sure helped. But, man, this clay! It's really made the noticeable difference in a fairly short time."

"That makes me feel a whole lot better, Al. How exactly do you use it?"

"I just slather it on my feet, and let it dry. I'll tell you something you might want to tell others. I think it does just as well, sometimes better, to just soak the feet in your clay water. You know, nice and hot. I'm sleeping so much better, and Joan even notices how much better I rest at night. My doctor is really impressed. Says he's coming out to see you. Doctor Ryan's a podiatrist in North Las Vegas. Has he been out?"

"Not that I know of, but of course, I'm not here all the time. And we're not really into using the clay on a serious basis. It's all new to us."

"Are you selling the stuff?"

"No, I wouldn't know what to charge. The old timers around here swear by it for all sorts of things. They're serious too! I'm going to have to learn a lot more about it before I start using the stuff to solve our health problems!" Al thought for a second and said, "You know what? I know you're gonna be careful, but nonetheless, I got a hunch you've found a new service of sorts. You like healing things, don't you?"

"Yeah, it's fun."

"Have you used this clay on arthritis before?"

"Nope, I haven't, but I'm getting ready to use it on a bunch of things, if what I think is true and if it checks out."

"How are you going to check it out?"

"Maybe at the University in Las Vegas. I imagine that they could tell me something."

"Cano, you might have a big deal. There's a lot of arthritis

78

around. I mean this stuff has helped me when nothing else did, and you'd have no shortage of customers. Doctor Ryan's office is always full. A lot of people in Las Vegas are on their feet all day and night. These puppies take a real beating. It's a big problem for a lot of folks in that town. I'd sure like to pay something and take enough home to last a while."

"No problem, Al, but keep your money in your pocket. You've made some good sense and opened my eyes. Anyway the stuff should be for free. I'll have the girl get some, wherever it is. Take all you want and let me know what all you use it for."

"That's great! I've got a couple of neighbors who can use it. I'll keep score on how we use it, and what happens. I figure we'll be coming back out sometime later next month."

"It's gonna be hot!" I said with a chuckle.

"Hey, Las Vegas is hot! All that concrete covering everything! Naw, this place is cool to us."

We both laughed at the joke. I liked his attitude. "Al, please tell your wife, if she'd like, we'll call a dentist in Pahrump for an appointment. No reason to go through that kind of pain! It's only a half-hour drive."

"Thanks, Cano. I enjoyed talking to you. I'll check on her. Before I leave, Cano, some of the guests were talking last night and mentioned that you wanted to build a–what you call–a Healing Center here on your place of some kind."

I nodded, "Yes."

"You're serious?"

"Yep! That's my general idea. It just seems a long way off sometimes, but yes. I'd love to create something, though I'm not sure what!"

Offering his hand, he encouraged me. "Well, keep at it. You build it and Las Vegas will come by the busloads. This area could be a tremendous place for a healing center, with the water and off the beaten path and all."

Al had to ask just one more question. "By the way, there's

something I want to ask you, do you have any relatives in Las Vegas?"

"I sure do, a brother." We both knew instantly that we were going in the same direction.

"He's a doctor? Right?"

"Yep, he's been there for several years."

" Dr. Frank, right?"

"Yep. He's my younger brother by eighteen months."

At that moment, Joan joined us on the patio. She took us by surprise with her clay-covered face.

She said, "Look at me Allan. This would cost me at least twenty-five dollars in town! It's great! You won't believe this stuff, this clay! Do you know what it's doing?"

Al interrupted her. "Hey, 'J' you won't believe this. Doc Frank is Cano's brother, his younger brother. Can you believe it?"

Joan went wide-eyed and her jaw dropped open, making her clay-covered face take on a comical look. Then she yelled, "No? Doctor Frank is your brother? What a small world."

Al said, "Tell me about it! Cano, what does your brother think about this clay?"

"Well, he doesn't know much, but then what doctor does? He's interested for sure. In fact, he's trying to figure how it can make him money."

"This is all too much, but get set for this. You're not going to believe me. I'm telling you guys, but when I started doing my facial with the clay I felt a pulling, a tightening kind of sensation, and get this, on my cheek over my bad tooth. Anyway, after it dried, I washed it all off and I applied the clay again. But then I put a glob of the clay directly over the tooth, just to see what would happen."

Al studied his wife. "I wondered what was up, and that's for the tooth? On the outside?"

Joan said excitedly, "Yes, I think I've invented something! See, the clay is still there and damp because it's thicker. Anyway,

80

it's pulling. I can feel it pulling around the tooth!"

Al asked, "What are you saying?"

"I'm saying that I can feel it pulling the infection out! I can feel it!"

"Oh come on, get outta here. Through the cheek?"

Joan insisted, "I know what you're thinking, Baby, but it feels that way!"

Al turned to me. "Cano, have you ever heard of this?"

I shook my head. "Nope, I've heard of it being used on the inside of the mouth, against infected gums or loose teeth, but never on the outside." Joan said, "Hey, you guys can imagine or not. It's my tooth. I'm telling you, it's been an hour-and-a-half, and my tooth is better. Look!" She ungraciously opened her mouth wide for Al to inspect it.

"Hell, I can't tell anything by looking. I didn't see it before." He glanced at me and said, "Too much! I'll take the girl's word for it."

She said emphatically, "Baby, I'm telling you it's better, and I'm leaving this stuff on no matter what until it dries. And then, I'm putting some more on. It's working! Understand? I mean, I was about to head to town. This thing was killing me."

Al surrendered. "Okay, okay. I got it. I don't see how, but I got it."

A proud and happy camper, I said, "Folks, this seems in order. Do either of you care for a chilled glass of white wine by any chance?"

Quickly, I had two takers. After going through a couple of rounds, I had a great idea. "Why don't we all go to dinner together? The diner in town has just been remodeled and the food's great. I'm buying."

Al said, "Sounds like a great idea."

As soon as we walked into the newly remodeled diner, Ruth Badame and Sylvia Burton spotted us and waved us over. They were sitting at a table for four and invited us to pull up another chair to join them. To my surprise, Al and Joan had known Ruthie and Sylvia for the several years.

Sylvia noticed Joan's face. "Joan, you've got clay on your face. Who did that?"

Joan, very proud of herself said, "I did it. I've invented a new way to cure tooth infections."

Ruthie said, "Joan, if your tooth is even a little sore, you'll love the clam chowder. It's Boston-style and as good as anything in Las Vegas."

Al smacked his lips. "Thanks, Ruthie, sounds good. Me too!"

At the end of the meal, I leaned over to Sylvia and whispered, "The clay on Joan's face didn't really surprise you for a tooth problem, did it? You know more than you let on, don't you? I saw you with the Hadleys, but there's a lot more, isn't there?"

Sylvia smiled and said coyly, "Yes, I do. And it's time we told you some things. How about coffee in the morning about 10:00 at my place? I'll invite Mori and possibly Art and Luella too." She looked at me intently and said, "You're ready for school, my boy. But come over early for breakfast, say 8:00? Your mom and I have decided something you should know about."

I couldn't resist the invitation. "I'll be there."

⚃ ⚃ ⚃

Sylvia fixed corned beef hash and eggs, my favorite. By now, the clock read past 9:00. School would begin in less than an hour. Helping to clean up the breakfast table, and drying the dishes for her reminded me of doing the same for Mom so many times. For a few minutes we didn't talk much, and just did the dishes.

Curious, I asked her, "What's this about you and mother that you think I should know?"

A soft smile started off in her eyes and spread to her shoulders. She fidgeted a little and began, "Well as you know, your mother and I have been talking about different things, and I was

82

telling her about my girls being way off, and about my son being killed in the accident and all. Anyway she told me that you said some nice things about me and, well, do you know what Eva suggested?"

Sylvia's question intrigued me. "I have no idea, but I think you're about to tell me, right?"

"Eva said to me, 'Well, Sylvia, why don't you be Cano's Second Mother? And he can be your second son!'"

She anticipated my heartfelt reaction and sweetened the moment. "I have something for you, one of your favorite things."

Getting up from the table she said, "I talked to Eva, and she told me about something you've enjoyed since you were a boy."

"Since I was a boy? Enjoyed?"

"She said you used to watch them for hours."

"Hmmm...girls?" I waited for a second then said, "Just kidding."

Sylvia playfully pointed her finger at me to say, "You'll see. I'll be right back."

She quickly returned from her bedroom carrying something covered with a lace doily. I thought to myself that whatever she carried had her features, old-fashioned lace and all. Holding her gift in one hand she held out the other and said, "Let's sit on the sofa. Bring your coffee."

She placed her lace-covered container on the coffee table and we sat down.

I sensed she had imagined us sitting just this way on her sofa when she gave me this gift.

She turned to me and said, "Cano, time passes so fast and sometimes we don't get to say the things we want to say, or do the things we want to do, for those we love. You know what I mean? I mean when we have a chance to?"

Her sweet words touched me deeply. All I could muster was, "Yes, I know."

She took my hand in both of hers, and affectionately

continued. "Dear, I don't get to see you everyday, or talk to you. But I want you to think of me every morning from now on. When you get up and start your day I want you to be reminded of me, and know that my prayers will always include you and Eva."

"Sylvia, that's so sweet of you."

She reached over to slip the lace off a beautiful cigar box shaped chest that looked like a pure Sylvia Burton creation. She meticulously constructed this little chest by covering the side surfaces with several hues of sand, and then on top of the sand tastefully fastened her collection of small, pebbles. Framing a stunning scene painted in miniature on the lid, she had mounted her collection of blue lapis, which she knew was my favorite stone.

The scene she painted on the lid was a sunrise scene as viewed from Tecopa Hot Springs looking east toward the mountains.

"Sylvia, you made this for me? I've never, I mean, this is the most beautiful gift I've ever received."

As I picked up the little chest I mumbled, "This is a treasure I'll keep forever." Partially opening the lid, I was spellbound by the sight of twelve exquisite crystals laid on a plush royal blue velvet lining. Speechless, I looked up at her smiling face. "Oh my God, Sylvia they're fabulous and so big!"

She reached over, picked one up and said, "If you'll notice they all have little eyelets so you can hang 'em over your windows."

"Yes, they're perfect!" I examined each one with a practiced eye and knew these would refract colored light beams all over the place like crazy! "Oh Sylvia, they're wonderful."

She said, "I understand you once had a crystal as a boy." I must have had an incredulous look on my face. She continued, "Your mom said you had one when you were eleven, and you played with it on a string in the morning sunlight." Then Sylvia laughed and said, "But you never told her where it came from."

"Nope! I wouldn't dare tell her. Whew! Never did and never will! My, my these are simply beautiful." Then I got up and put my treasure on her table for all to see.

Sylvia went to the kitchen to make a fresh pot of coffee and get some pastries ready when she began to tell a story that soon had me in stitches. She was going through an animated description of a pious young preacher who was to deliver a guest sermon at the new local church one Sunday morning back in the early 40s.

"He was in the process of demonstrating his manliness, combined with an exhibition of the milk of human kindness." She tried to put off the thought by waving her hands as though through invisible smoke. Then, she returned to the drama. "Cano, he was doing all this by rescuing a local tom cat from a tree beside the church. The old cat had again retreated to safety of the tree in order to avoid his dreaded enemy, Dusty, a very busy local dog."

It wasn't like Sylvia to be so expressive when she talked, but this morning she was quite animated. I leaned back in the sofa and opened my ears for her delightful story.

"Well, the old cat didn't find the scene at all amusing. He wasn't meowing to get down or anything, and he knew the situation only too well. He was mad, and now this city-boy preacher decides to save this mean ole` tom, right?" She rolled her eyes to indicate the futility of the idea. "Allen, the preacher got a chair from the church and with a great show of bravado reached up to grab the old tom. Several of us wondered if he had any idea what he was doing.

"Then Allen said, 'Here Kitty, Kitty. Nice kitty,' and then he extended himself on tiptoes as he lunged for the cat's neck."

I had fun just watching Sylvia tell her story. "When the bright young preacher had stretched full out, and with searching fingers getting far too close to his nose, the chewed up old tom met him half way by pouncing on the preacher's bare arm."

Sylvia found her own story hilarious. "Then that cat got extremely busy clawing with all four paws digging, scraping and slashing, as if that arm was Dusty."

I had to laugh as she vividly recounted the story.

Sylvia didn't let up. "Cano, this sweet young preacher desperately hung onto a limb with one hand. The kitty was all over the free arm, and the chair was on its side, kicked out from under the man by his thrashing legs."

Sylvia, now seated and with both hands covering her face, continued to laugh. I had never heard her laugh so fully. She hadn't even thought of this story in, I wondered how many years.

She regained her poise, winked and said, "Son, now I don't mean to make too much fun of our young preacher's plight but he was a sight, sitting on the ground bewildered by the unexpected fury of it all."

I came off the sofa and gave her a big hug. "Sylvia, what a story! I loved it!"

"You should hear Beulah tell it! See, Cano, Allen was staying with Beulah and Harry. Harry wanted their guest to spread a solution of clay on the arm immediately to control the bleeding and clean the wounds, especially to stop any infection. That was the real danger from the old tom's scratches.

"You see, Beulah's husband had a lot of experience because of his men on the railroad getting banged up and dealing with infections all the time. They were a long way from a doctor out there and Harry knew what the clay could do. Anyway, the preacher wouldn't have any of it, pure city boy. He said he'd be okay, no problem. In a show of grandiose posturing he said for all the crowd to hear that he'd just wash-up and <u>pray</u> on it." Sylvia glanced out the front window and said, "Here they come!"

"Who?" I said.

"Art and Luella. I can hear 'em in their old van a block away."

I wanted her to finish the story, "So what happened to the preacher man?"

"Well, Beulah's husband was sort of crusty at times. Anyway, he just shrugged his shoulder indifferently and said, 'Al, it's up to you, but I'd put clay on that arm and I'd do it now. That's a nasty old cat."

I pictured the scene and smiled to myself when I thought, the young preacher had denied the God-given power of our clay and trusted his uninformed youthful judgment. On the other hand the same God had endowed, and in fact blessed the old tom with some God-given claws to keep fools at bay.

I was still smiling as Sylvia continued fixing the pastries. "Anyway, the next morning, the young man's arm looked really bad, terribly swollen and severely infected. Beulah's husband, still seemingly indifferent asked, 'Okay, Pastor, what do you want to do? Do you want me to drive you for two hours to the hospital, and not accomplish what the clay can do or what?"

Allen said, "Harry, I've prayed on it and the Lord says I should use the clay."

Harry looked him over and said, "Me and the Lord agree."

The van doors were slamming shut.

She had me. "Whatever happened to him, the preacher?"

My new mom said, "Oh, he healed up fine, went back to Los Angeles and kept preaching. He's retired now and lives in Santa Monica. He doesn't come here often. He likes the ocean a lot better."

"Do you know him?"

"Sure, he's my little brother."

I came off the sofa. "Are you kidding me?"

At that moment, Art banged on the door with his usual gusto.

Sylvia yelled, "Come on in! Before you break my door!"

They were an impressive threesome. Art appeared as though ready to hunt bear. Luella presented the classic picture of a 1910 schoolteacher in a long dress with bonnet and carrying a satchel of papers. Last in the door stepped Mori, sporting a completely wild purple beret that gave him the air of a small Frenchman on a huge mission.

Art noticed the chest first. "When did you make this Sylvia? The border of blue lapis really sets it off."

Luella and Mori were examining the work when Art lifted the

lid and saw the crystals. "Good grief! Look here, Lou. It's like a treasure chest of crystals!"

"I made it for Cano." Sylvia cocked her head. "He likes to play with crystals." Then she welcomed them, "Make yourself comfortable. Care for some coffee and a sweet roll?"

Art was ready.

She started to laugh again. "Oh my, I was just telling Cano about the time Allen and the old tom cat got tangled up in the tree."

Art smiled at the memory of the story. "I've heard that story from several people. Wish I'd been there to see it. I sure miss all the good stuff."

Mori said, "You should hear Beulah tell the story. It gets better every year. By the way, how's Allen? Is he still in L.A.?"

Sylvia replied, "Yes, Yes. Bless his heart." She began to serve coffee and some of her special Danish. Sylvia broke up again when she added, "And he still doesn't like cats."

Mori broke the levity by proclaiming in his best business manner, "Now then Cano, are you ready for a course of Clay Therapy 101?"

I nodded emphatically. "Professor, bring it on!"

The big little man carefully removed his beret, gently placed it on the table, looked slowly around the room as if to recheck that everything was in order, and broke into a smile. "Fine. Let's begin."

Art headed for their van to get Lou's blackboard for Mori. "Did you remember the colored chalk?" He glanced over his shoulder and repeated somewhat louder, "Lou, did you remember the..."

Lou tried to quiet Art. "Hush! Yes! Yes, it's in the box behind the seat, and bring in the eraser." She turned to Sylvia and asked, "Can Mori use one of your easels to put the blackboard on?"

"Oh, sure. That'll work perfect. I'll get the big one."

Mori systematically fumbled through his antiquated brief case.

I grinned to myself and figured he hadn't had a cause to use that well-worn relic in perhaps thirty years. This morning the beautiful but tattered old leather case was like a time traveler, carrying him back to the hectic university life he had left long ago. The dear man was contentedly engrossed while the four of us were as curious as his students of yesteryear while he searched each compartment; deftly extracting a particular sheet, examined it briefly, and placed it carefully in his working folder.

Finally aware of his audience, he gently closed his folder, tapped it on the table as if to say, "I'm ready," and under his breath whispered, "Brevity. One must remember brevity."

He pushed himself from the table and with the work folder in his left hand acting as a fan, strode to the blackboard. He picked up a fresh stick of green chalk and printed at the top of the board in six-inch letters the title of his presentation.

CALCIUM BENTONITE

Therapeutic Clay: History and Uses

He pointed to the blackboard. "You see that I've given our clay a name which reflects where it is and what it is. For brevity, let's call it TC. All right, we've got a lot of material to cover, but I believe you'll find this subject extremely interesting and informative.

"As we know the topic isn't completely foreign to us. A few of us have been using it to some degree for some time." Turning to me he said, "Certainly, I've uncovered enough for you to realize that our particular clay isn't merely a local phenomena or folklore-type thing, as you once described it.

"Cano, what I'm laying out for you is an outline of the subject using pertinent points. I've got this all typed and arranged so that you don't have to take any specific notes unless you have questions."

I nodded.

"You know, many of us around here shouldn't have to plead guilty because we're somewhat uninformed regarding the dimensions of this subject. I'd bet a dinner in Las Vegas that not one physician in a thousand has any concept of clay therapy. This in spite of the recorded facts by the greatest names in medicine for hundreds of years that have firmly established the fundamental medical integrity of certain clays."

He wrote on the board, History, and said, "I've got pages of material dealing with the history of the subject. I'm talking about all over Europe, China, South America, Africa. By the way, slaves were the ones who really popularized the use of clay in the South. Of course, Indians all over North and South America have used it forever for internal and external use."

He handed the papers to me. "Go over this so you'll be completely up to speed and understand how widespread it is."

"Oh, I will. This is a big win for me already." I addressed everyone when I said, "Rest assured that for me to know that clay therapy has a dignified and sophisticated history is a big, big deal. I didn't expect this. I didn't know that there was anything printed on this subject."

"And, Cano, I promise, my boy, you ain't seen nothing yet!"

Art said, "Sic `em, Mori!" Everyone burst into laughter.

"I can't wait. This is interesting stuff, but you know, when I look over my notes of how I've personally used the clay, along with what I've seen and heard about this medical use for clay. Well, it has a science fiction flavor to it."

Mori jumped at my analogy. "Yes! Yes! You got it! But what you also have acquired within the Science Fiction description is a problem, a serious problem with communication. Science Fiction? Good way to view it! But this Science Fiction stuff is real. No matter that it really works in multiple ways, that's a fact, but that's not the issue! The true issue to be concerned about is that for seventy-five years, since World War One, and for sure after World

War Two, Mr. and Mrs. America have been saturated and conditioned with drugs of all sizes and shapes for everything imaginable. And clay therapy, no matter how effective, is very different from what everyone is used to. And that's a communication problem." Art, as anxious as the rest of us, asked, "Okay, so how does the stuff work?"

I said, "Thanks, Art. That nails it down. Mori, what is it doing, and why is it doing whatever it's doing? I've seen some unusual results. I mean this clay makes me look like a healer. Hell, I'm no healer. A monkey could put our clay on someone, and it would work!"

Mori nodded in agreement. "Cano, you don't know how right you are." He picked up a sheet of paper, and showed it to us.

"Some of the really great therapeutic clay deposits have been found by following injured animals. That fact was known hundreds of years ago, but let's move on."

He cleared the board and seemed more serious than usual when he asked, "Does anyone know what the cells in our body feed on? And does anyone know what our clay is made of?"

At this moment, Mori's demeanor grew more intense as he got to a serious point in his presentation. He used blue chalk to print:

<u>Nourishment for Cells:</u> Trace Minerals
Our Clay is: <u>100% Trace Minerals</u>

He turned to look at us and said, "What I'm saying is that our clay consists of 100% trace minerals and these trace minerals provide the micronutrients for every cell in the body."

No one said a word. We all knew that we had just heard some heavy stuff.

"Cano, you might take a look at this and pass it around. Thanks to Luella, some students at UNLV did an analysis of the clay for us."

I scanned the paper: Silicon (SiO_2) 34%; Calcium (CaO) 21%; Krypton (K_2O) 5.35% Magnesium (MgO) 16%; Sodium (Na_2O)

4.2%; Aluminum (Al_2O_3) 10.93671%; Titanium (TiO_2) 8.2%; Boron (B_2O_3) 0.098%; Manganese (MnO)0.036%; Iron (Fe_2O_3) o.036%; Gallium (Ga_2O_3) 0.0046%; Cobalt (C_0O) 0.001% (TRO); Copper (Cu0) 0.0033%; Nickel (NiO) 0.00019%; Vanadium (V_2O_5) 0.013%; Strontium (SrO) 0; Chromium (Cr_2O_3) 0.0012%; Other Elements-NIL. Mori continued. "I find it fascinating that when you examine the breakdown, you realize that the mineral breakdown is similar to the breakdown of trace minerals in the human body! For instance, about 20% of the minerals in our body are calcium and about 20% of the clay is—you got it—*calcium*! But let's move on. We have lots of ground to cover. Excuse the pun."

We all groaned. He wrote.

How Does Clay Work?

While we read the analysis of our clay, Mori continued. "The answer to this question strikes at the heart and defines the difference between Alopathic-Pharmaceutical medicine and Therapeutic clay. First, we need to understand that this clay works safely and executes several different functions at the same time, unlike usual pharmaceuticals.

"Let me put it as simply as I can. Drugs, any drugs are chemical agents. They're powerful as a treatment, but can be equally dangerous in terms of side effects. This clay works in an entirely different manner. Clay, as a natural physical agent has no side effects. Our therapeutic clay uses electromagnetic action, a physical action rather than a chemical one."

I leaned forward in my chair when he started to discuss this intriguing subject.

"Remarkably, our clay has a constant negative electrical attraction for all kinds of debris or areas of the body with a positive charge. Just to name a few, I found that chemicals, inflammation, infection, fungus, 'bad' bacteria, pain, or torn tissue in the system all have negative charges." Then he wrote: "And *all* are *irresistibly* drawn towards the clay." He appeared fox-like when he said, "Additionally, restricted capillaries in the head that cause migraines are positive. The clay seems to relax the positive trauma and lets the blood flow."

Confused, I closed my eyes and began massaging my temples. "Mori, by that definition the clay would work on the majority of common day to day medical problems. If that's what you're saying, it's a bit much to swallow. . Who would ever believe it? I mean, talk about Science Fiction." I stretched both arms overhead and said half-joking, "If they found something like what you're talking about on the moon, hell, they'd have space ships going after it!"

Art said, "Mori, do you mean that..."

Mori stopped the crosstalk. "I'm saying that from what I've learned so far, and you haven't heard it all yet, that - Yes, Cano - you may in the future have a problem in telling the whole clay story because of the multiple therapeutic action use of this particular clay. Remember the pharmaceuticals. Beware!"

"Are you telling me that if we start showing too many people how to treat and heal themselves that I'll have legal problems?" I thought, as if my Biz isn't tough enough, now I'm gonna have to worry about clay.

As Mori approached the blackboard he turned and said, "Times are changing, Cano, people are tired of the status quo in health care. People want something different, Holistic Medicine."

Luella, Art, and Sylvia nodded their agreement.

Mori motioned to his blackboard. "You see listed Absorbent-Adsorbent-Physics-Catalyst, and so forth. These subjects will allow me to dive into the guts of our story, and I'll do this with a general discussion. Remember, we know that the clay is a negatively charged substance. When taken internally or applied externally, the miniscule clay particles permeate throughout the system down to the cellular level."

Art asked, "It goes right through the skin?"

"Quicker than you can get to fried chicken!"

Luella laughed. "That was a good one, Mori."

Mori smiled. "I don't want to get too technical today, but this part touches on the physics of the question." To make the next point Mori uncovered a saucer of our gray-greenish powdered clay and with a wooden tongue depressor began playing with the powder by scooping up some on the depressor, and pouring back into the saucer. "To appreciate the whole subject, one needs to know that the basic physics of the stuff is mind boggling. The very size and shape of each infinitesimally small negatively charged particle of the clay is astounding. Each rectangular particle is not only unbelievably small but also extremely flat relative to its mass. This whole magnetic property that this clay possesses wouldn't or couldn't happen if the shape wasn't as I've described." Sylvia looked over the glasses perched on her nose. "This is nothing, Mori, but I'm curious. You said real small, compared to what? How small and why is that important?"

Mori picked up and poured streams of clay with his depressor and contemplated Sylvia's question.

Sylvia said, "Sorry, Mori. I didn't mean to interrupt."

He said, "Oh no, not at all, dear. It's really a very interesting point, both the question and the answer. You see this particular type of green clay has particles so minute that it was calculated by some guy at MIT that if one could lay out flat, side by side, one gram of this substance, it would cover 800 square meters! That would make each particle smaller than smoke!"

Art said, "Oh, come on, Mori! Smoke?"

"I'm telling you, Art. One gram would equal 800 square meters."

Luella "the thinker" paused a moment from her note taking. "I don't understand. It's impressive, but why is it so important?"

Mori rose to the moment. "Ah yes. Now, we have a question. Why?" He moved like a fighter with an opening and with yellow chalk as his weapon he printed in big perfect letters:

94

Absorption/Adsorption

"The term that science uses to describe what the clay does when it gets close to a positively-charged particle in the tissue of the body is Absorption. Our clay does the same thing in the body's fluid such as blood, bile, and lymph glands by adsorption."

I took a note when he said, "This quality clay acts like a scavenger in the blood. The clay never stops hunting for debris. It acts like a blood purifier."

Art stood up, stretched all of his 250 pounds, and said, "Well, I'll be dad gum. You mean it works that way on everything?"

Mori decided to sit down, and took a deep breath. "Well, yes. It does other important things in the body, but, yes, generally it works that way. You know it seems to me that our clay acts like a referee, getting all the bad positively-charged stuff out of the way so the body can heal itself."

Art said, "That makes a lot of sense but there's something I don't get. For years..."

Luella stopped Art. "Mori, have you had enough today? You've been going steady for some time."

"Thanks but I'm fine. I'll just sit for a while. We don't have too much further to go. Now, Art, what don't you get?"

Art said, "Luella's sister has used our clay for years on her migraines. I always figured it was just a...what do they call it when you think it's gonna work, and it does? Lou, what do they call it?"

"Placebo, dear. It's called the placebo effect," Luella said.

"Yes. That's it. Placebo."

Mori asked, "Just how does she use it?"

"Just puts a wet wash cloth soaked in clay over her face. I've seen her. We've seen her, huh Lou? Leaves it on for about a half-hour."

Lou agreed.

Mori said, "You know, folks, when I reviewed all the material,

I got to thinking and came up with an explanation of why it works. The clay particles go to wherever there's a need in the body because this stuff works by electromagnetic attraction! If Lou's sister has a migraine and the capillaries are restricted and positively-charged and cutting off the blood flow, which is causing the migraine, and the clay is magnetically attracted to that spot, then the clay neutralizes and relaxes the capillaries and allows the blood to flow. Well, that could be the answer as to why and how it works."

"Well, I'll be darned. Okay. Here's another one. I saw it used 35 years ago by an Indian. Oh, Luella, what's his name, the Shoshone from Death Valley? Had his foot broke real good?"

"That's Sue's boy, Harold."

"Yes, that's it. He was down by the horseshoe pit with his foot all broke and puffed up cause a truck had backed over it. Anyway, it was bad, but he wouldn't go to town. He was sorta drunk. So that miner, Red, oh, what's his name? You know the big good-looking guy. Used to work with Beulah's husband. Anyway, Red packed his foot in clay. It took all night to dry, but the next morning, I heard that he woke up and they said you couldn't tell no difference between his feet. The foot was still broke-up, but it wasn't swollen!

"Harold was all the time getting drunk and hurting himself. He was lucky to be down there when he did it, and he was lucky Red was in the Snake Pit."

Mori broke in. "I'd never heard that story. Boy, the Snake Pit has a lot of 'em."

Sylvia said, "I heard it, the story. I was there, or here. Red got the clay from me that night. In fact, Harold slept back there on the porch. You know as I recall, he never went to the doctor. No need to. It was healing just fine. I remember some guys made a clay cast for him to keep it from moving around. He used to bathe his foot in the water and put clay in it. Did that for a couple of weeks. Harold finally quit drinking and lives in Barstow now. Retired from the county."

I said, "Sylvia, that's a heck of a story."

She said, "Nice memories, too. Red was my fella for some time back then."

Mori stared at Sylvia incredulously. "That's remarkable. I read where it's very effective in cases of a sprain or swelling, but a broken foot? Now, I remember Red, big guy must have been 6'4". You two used to dance a lot and had a few squabbles if I remember."

Sylvia said, "Yes. It's all true." And then smiling said, "Making up was the best part."

Art tactfully ignored the last statement and moved on. "One more and I'm finished. I never saw it work on a burn, but remember when Sylvia put it on that man, Hadley, on the burnt arm, a couple of months back? That wasn't the same as a sprain or food poisoning or some infection that was going crazy. That was a burn. Now, how can you account for all we know and heal a burn too?"

For a long moment the significance and complexity of Art's question hung in the air.

Mori's bemused expression turned to awe. "A screaming nerve ending has a positive charge. The clay locks onto it, protects it from infection, and stops the pain. This stuff is God's referee alright." He held his hands out in a pleading fashion. "Blows me away."

Though none of us had any medical training, as if touched by a magic wand, all the loose data gelled into a functional structure of its own. Now we knew. From then on we recognized that the value to so many, the inherent responsibility within this moment, weighed heavily upon us.

Mori spoke softly. "The clay has almost a mystical feature. It's wonderful stuff. God-given. It supports, sustains, and defends the living body as though directed by the Creator. I have some more information here." We had never seen Mori so moved. He opened his lovely old case one more time and produced a sheet of paper and said, "I copied this from the work of an internationally recognized clay physician, a researcher from France, Raymond Dextreit. Let me share his conclusions with you."

Mori read solemnly from the paper.

"One of green clay's peculiarities is based on its electro physical domination. From a thermodynamic point of view, we must admit that certain types of gray-green clay cannot be the sole energy of the phenomena it produces. This clay is effective through a dynamic presence far more significant than a mere consideration of the substances it contains. It's a catalyst rather than an agent in itself. This is possible because clay is alive; 'living earth.'"

Mori removed his beret and sat down, satisfied. The four of us just sat there for a few seconds and looked at our dear friend. He had just given his best. Sylvia started and the rest followed with a gentle applause.

Time For A Walk

In her inimitable style, Ruthie prepared a lovely dinner that evening complete with bringing the dishes and silverware. Beulah didn't have the strength to attend the day-long session, but she wanted to enjoy dinner with us. In keeping with her matriarch status that she had filled for so many years, the lady simply wanted to know what had transpired in her absence.

Art said, "Beats the daylights outta me–all the things our clay does, especially the fact that there's so much in books about it." He looked to his friend. "Beulah, do you know what they call it when they're treating folks with clay? There's a name for it!"

"I didn't know there was any such name. We just used to call it the Healin' Mud."

Art went on. "Well, we've all been right about that, but the name was wrong. We named it for what it did. Science gave it a name for what it is. Seems like the Greeks gave us a name for everything, including the clay. They called it *Pelotherapy*. Ha! We call it Tecopa's Therapeutic Clay."

"Sounds like you've done a lot of research."

"Oh, it's been a good learning day. Real good."

Mori sat unusually quiet, which drew further attention to the professional way he had accomplished his task.

Beulah asked, "Well, Mr. Instructor, how did it go? Are you satisfied? It looks like you have some excited students."

Mori first looked at Beulah, and then the rest. "We all learned a lot today." Then after glancing at me for a second, smiled ever so slightly. "Far more than we anticipated."

I looked at Beulah, smiled, and confirmed what Mori had said, "Yes. Far more. I've got a great deal to assimilate. This brings my education to a head."

Sylvia said, "Well son, so you think you've learned enough?"

I said, "Ruthie, the dinner was great. Beulah, you can be proud of your friends for all these years. They did a heck of a job." I stood up and walked over to Art. "I'm glad you're here big guy. Lord knows we need you." Then I kissed Luella on the cheek and said, "Thanks so much."

Lou replied, "It was our pleasure."

When I approached Mori, he appeared completely satisfied. I started to shake his hand, and then hugged him again. "You're too much."

Then to Sylvia, "Well, Mom, it was a fine day."

She looked so happy, "We all love ya', Son."

I gathered up my notes and papers. "Heck of a day. I'll never forget, never. I'm blessed. This community is blessed to have you all. I'm gonna go now. I told Mom I'd call and I want to take a walk, a long walk."

Beulah said, "Cano, tell Little Eva we love her and to come visit us soon." She had given her stamp of approval.

"I sure will."

Close to the door I turned and said, "You all know how I feel about the way you've treated me and Mom."

Luella spoke up, "We know. Go call Eva, and take a long walk."

As soon as I got to my place, I tried to call Mom, but she wasn't home. I decided to catch her later. For now, I wanted to take a hot bath and a swim before I took my walk. By the time I got through with both it was evening, just before sundown. I chose my favorite walking staff, picked up a half full bottle of Bailey's, a fat roach, and started walking and thinking. I walked straight East.

No one ever walked straight East into the desert out there. There was no path, just gullies and dunes. After awhile I realized I was in an area that I hadn't been in before. It was neat. I could talk to myself. I could cry. I could yell my guts out, and the sand and sky would soak up everything.

The questions that had bugged me for the last few months swirled around my head. How could the remarkable deposit of clay exist without being marketed or at least used as a companion to the mineral water to create a valid and desperately needed new service?

How could Tecopa Hot Springs exist, broken down or not, with the clean fresh hot mineral water, and with what looked like a world-class deposit of therapeutic clay, along with desert clean air, hundreds of inexpensive acres to build on, and all of this an hour or so from Las Vegas, Nevada?

To top it off it's all next to the awe-inspiring major resort of Death Valley, an hour's drive from Baker, California, and one of the busiest freeways in the world between Los Angeles and Las Vegas!

I couldn't fathom why some of the smartest, most innovative, aggressive and far-sighted business people in the world, those who created Las Vegas, hadn't already snapped up every square inch in the area, and develop it into some sort of health center for the million plus citizens who lived in Las Vegas alone. Not to mention the draw of a very different type of a holistically-oriented, recreational, cultural community that could service the swarm of 30,000,000 tourists who invade the area yearly.

After tripping on these points again, I got up and shouted, "To hell with what I don't understand. To hell with trying to figure out why *they* don't paint this canvas the way it was meant to be. Screw it! I'm gonna do it for 'em. Frank Lloyd Wright, I'm not, but he said, 'Form Follows Function.' He said it. I believe it, and that's that."

I was standing on the top of the highest dune and yelling, "This is a healing, recreational, cultural community!" I shouted louder. "The base of which is hot mineral water and the finest grade of therapeutic clay in the world! And a perfect lo-ca-tion!"

Exhausted from the complete catharsis, I flopped down, lay back in the warm sand, took a few hits and sips and laughed with the stars. I was a happy man. I had found something I wanted to do, a lot to do. I talked to the stars, "I have a purpose, and I know what I'm supposed to do!"

As I lay there the strange quote from Emerson flooded out my other thoughts, "The efforts which we make to escape our Destiny only serve to lead us into it."

A twister for me, I decided this whip-like thought was Emerson's way of relating the importance of choices. I had to call Mom.

Chapter 9

Curt Hibdon: A Class Act

Fate makes our relatives; Choice makes our friends.

Jacques DeLille

The sound of Curt Hibdon's tractor woke me before sunrise. With a cup of coffee in hand, I watched him through my front window as he leveled a part of Delight's land. He was moving a lot of dirt. He worked like a chess player, anticipating moves long before they came up. Curt reminded me of an artist who could see his task complete and avoided costly mistakes.

Ruthie loved bringing me together with people she thought I should know. Promptly at 11:45 she and Curt arrived at my door.

She said, "Cano Graham, this is Curt Hibdon."

We shook hands.

He had unusually stout thick hands with a soft thoughtful grip. Heavy-set, probably 230 pounds, he had light skin with a ruddy complexion, light blue eyes and thinning, copper-colored hair. Quiet by nature, he gave the impression that he was shy.

I liked him the moment we met. Actually, I was looking forward to meeting him just by observing him on the tractor. "I didn't see you take a break all morning."

He looked at me curiously, then smiled slightly. "Oh, I just wanted to finish up before lunch. I told Delights that it would only be a half-day job." Then as I was to learn about him, he shifted the conversation away from himself. "You sure have done a good job cleaning this place up. It was a real mess."

"Thanks, Curt. I'm just trying to see what the canvas looks like. I've got a long way to go."

"Ruthie tells me you want to build a healin' place?" He appeared genuinely interested.

I said, "Well, that's a good description. I've been told that if I could think it, you could build it."

He looked at Ruthie for a moment to confirm where that opinion came from. "Well, yes-ah-thanks, Ruthie." And then back to me he said, "I do enjoy building things."

And so began the four-year creative run for Curt Hibdon and myself. If I could think it, he could build it. The two words I used to love to hear him say most were, "That'll work!"

I'd usually start off by saying, "Curt, I've got an idea."

He'd always stop whatever he was doing and say, "Well now, let's talk about it."

He had the habit of examining whatever idea I had, large or small, and after a long moment would either make a valid suggestion, question for clarification, or simply say, "That'll work!" Before too long we got real busy. I thought and he built. I had several tasks going on at the same time. I traveled a lot. Mom needed attention. And Curt or I constantly made trips to Las Vegas for supplies. Curt Hibdon handled thousands and thousands of dollars for me and always gave me an accounting to the penny.

I went through a lot of cash for supplies, equipment, payroll, and what have you, and Curt never once asked where the money came from.

Curt taught me that most workers don't know how to work. Our local help, not really used to working, held him in awe. His physical strength was legendary. He could lift a full 55-gallon drum on to a truck bed. One day I saw him stop the dozer when he was working on some rough rock. He got off shaking his hand, walked over to a clay pool, and put his hand into the clay. Then he wrapped his forefinger with a piece of clay-soaked cloth, and immediately resumed work.

After work I heard him tell Joyce, "You know our clay sure does work well. Stops pain real quick."

Two days later I found out he had broken his finger. I never heard him utter a word about it.

Chapter 10

Jamie

Each friend represents a world in us, a world possibly not born until they arrive, and it is only by this meeting that a new world is born.
Anais Nin

I hadn't been in the broken-down but beautiful little community very long, a couple of months or so, but long enough to upset the established rhythm of things. The first thing I did wrong was to talk about what I intended to do. Before long my workers were spending money at the store, and the bar was going strong. I loved the action, but some didn't love me, or all the new interest in town.

One Saturday afternoon, six of us sat at a big table, drinking and carrying on. The bar was full and we all sensed a new spirit in town. The music blared and the lights dimmed. We all had a certain buzz in our heads from the beer and the something new. Everyone knew that a big change was coming for Tecopa, California. For no apparent reason it got quiet in the room, except for our table. We all heard a chair being kicked, and everyone else sensed something. I was so new that I couldn't tell the standard from the unusual. They all glanced at me, then over my shoulder where the chair kicking took place.

There he stood in all his glory. He took the stance of a gunfighter, positioning himself for a shoot-out. He seemed tired for his age, and he looked as if he mustered all his courage to kick that chair. He began weaving a bit, and blinking slowly. Yelling with all the conviction that any tired soul motivated by beer could put together, "Cano!"

I turned my head in his direction. He seemed sort of taken aback by his own voice and the fact that he was on center stage.

"Yes?" I stared at him.

"I don't like you, or what you're doing."

I stayed in my chair and half-turned toward him. I nodded my head in a way that indicated I understood exactly what he meant. "Aren't you Jamie?"

Assuming the stance and attitude of a poor man's Billy the Kid, he courageously uttered, "I sure am."

"You know, Jamie? All my life, since I was a little boy, some people just naturally don't like me. I get along with most people okay, but *damn!* Every now and then I run into someone who just simply doesn't like me, and it never gets better. I admire you for speaking your piece, but don't feel bad about it. It's just natural for some to feel that way. So I won't worry about it if you don't, and maybe next time we'll get acquainted a little better, and we can find some common ground." Someone had already told me about Jaime and his interests. "By the way, I like animals. Do you?"

Unsteady and confused, he yelled, "Yeah, I like *little* animals."

I said, "Well, that's a start. Why don't I buy a fresh pitcher of beer, and talk about this later, I want to visit with my friends right now."

Bless his heart, he said, "Well, okay. I didn't know you liked animals."

Someone slapped him on the shoulder as if to say, "You did it Jamie...now let's have a beer."

Early one Monday morning, Jamie stood in the middle of the road waving his arms to flag me down. The sun glistened off his hair like a reflector. He knew it was my day to go to Las Vegas, but this wasn't like him to stop me. I eased to a stop.

"Morning, Cano." He was serious about something.

"Hi, Jamie. What's up?"

"Cano, do you think the clay would work on a mouse?"

I gave him a blank stare. "A mouse?"

"It's like this. You see my cat brought this mouse to me as a gift. You know how cats do that sort of thing."

He spoke to me as if he were giving me a lesson on the behavior of desert cats. "Yeah, I've seen that sort of thing. But usually the gift is dead, or near dead."

He corrected me. "Not always. This mouse has a bad cut on its leg, a recent cut. The cat didn't do it. He just brought it to me. What d'ya think?"

I felt like I was in a scene in a play I couldn't get out of. Then I realized I didn't want to get out. "I've never seen my clay fail to heal a wound, no matter where it is, or what it's on, or when it happened. Is the mouse at the house?"

"Nooo!" He replied like he had a bull in the pen waiting for the matador. He motioned me over to a box under his tree. He knew that I'd never leave to go anywhere without taking my clay with me. "You got it, don't you?"

"Sure. Let's look at this injury." It was just like he said, a big mouse with a nasty cut. I put some gloves on, picked him up so the leg wound was exposed, and smeared clay into it.

Jamie asked, "Done deal?"

"Yep, done deal. Let me know how this looks tomorrow."

"Sure enough."

As I got back in my truck Jamie said, "Cano, you know me and Betty haven't been getting on too good lately."

"I know, Jamie. I've talked to her about it. The drinking is kind of getting to her."

With his booted foot, he unconsciously shoved the sand into little piles, then pushed them away. He didn't look up when he said, "I know how she feels. Do you think I could get a couple days work this week?"

When he spent too much time in the bar, it was hard for Jamie to work because the heat just got to him. He wasn't afraid to work, he'd worked hard all his life, but the heat just got to him. He was kind of old for his age.

"Sure, Jamie, go see Curt. I'll tell him you're going to be helping out for a few days. We're starting early, you know."

"I'll be ready." The plot unfolded when he asked, "And by the way, do you think I might get a little advance on my wages? I'm kinda short."

"No problem, Jamie. Go easy, and get some rest tonight."

He was inspired. "I'll be ready. See you later, and drive safe, Cano. You know those wild horses are on the highway sometimes in the morning."

Jamie was something. He was going to have a fine day.

CB   CB   CB

Someone knocked on my door at 3:00 a.m. I had had a long day in Las Vegas. I had too much wine, and smoked some very tasty herb in Mountain Springs before I enjoyed a slow late night drive home under a friendly moon.

The banging continued. "Damn! Someone is serious!" I flipped the porch light on and opened the door. I couldn't see anything but a bloody, blonde head. Jamie stood with his head bowed and his shoulders slumped. I couldn't see his face. He raised his head finally, but I still couldn't make out his features for all the blood covering them.

I said, "Jamie, what in the hell?"

He interrupted me. "Betty hit me a bunch of times with a big iron frying pan." Jamie's day had been a full one, but things had started to fall apart when he arrived home late. He opened his sky blue eyes, and a big smile creased his weathered features. It seemed as if every inch of his face was covered with blood except

108

for his eyes and teeth. "But you know what, Cano? She loves me. Betty *really* loves me."

Then he sort of dropped his head and swayed from side to side. "She just got kind of carried away when I tried to show her how Martha was doing so much better and all. I mean Cano, she started to get that look, you know? But the real problem started when she saw me kiss Martha, and then tried to kiss her too. Women!"

"Jamie, what the hell are you talking about? I know Betty loves you, but who's Martha?"

He wiped some blood off his face. "I named her after Paul's wife, Martha. Don't you think it fits?"

I finally woke up. "Named who?"

The flash flood grew to a rolling torrent, and spilled over his lips. "My sweet little mouse. You wouldn't believe how much better her leg is, since just this morning! She's started moving around, and she's feeling a lot better."

The moon was hanging low, and so was my head. I remember thinking, "I can't be on Candid Camera. Is this really happening, or is this a dream?"

Jamie had won, and I was drained by it all. Betty was probably sleeping peacefully by now. Martha was peachy, and for a second I wondered about her leg, but I was limp and just couldn't absorb anymore. Then I whispered, as if talking in a normal tone of voice would get him started again, "Jamie, go to the outside shower and wash the blood off your head."

He blinked slowly, his eyes sticky with blood and exhaustion. With his jaw hanging a bit, he asked, "Don't you want to see her?"

"Jamie, I'm sure Betty will be fine. You didn't hit her, did you?"

"Betty? I'm not talking about Betty. I'm talking about Martha, my little Martha."

I swear I thought he was going to dissolve into tears. "The mouse! It's after three a.m. and you want me to see your mouse? I can't believe that you…What are you doing, Jamie?"

He was on a roll, a roll through my psyche, and he had a determined look in his eyes.

"I've got her right here." He pulled a rag from his pocket. With the wad of rag in his palm, he began to carefully uncover Martha. With great deliberation, he executed his task, and there was Martha!

Why is it that mice always appear to look directly at you? Martha was no different and was obviously staring at me. I cut off the thought before it had time to gain any substance.

"Put Martha back in your pocket, and go wash your head. Please, Jamie? Please?"

The laceration on Jamie's head was more than a cut. His scalp was smashed open a quarter-inch deep and a quarter-inch wide, running back from his hairline in a zigzag pattern about four to five inches in length. I clipped his hair with a pair of scissors along the lines of the laceration.

I clipped the hair as short as I could, and patted it dry. I poured dry powdered clay directly into the laceration, and then covered the entire area with gelled clay. I wiped off the excess, and told him not to touch it for any reason until it had dried completely.

I told him to keep applying the clay daily until the cut healed. Jamie had heard me say to get the clay on the injured area as quickly as possible and I had the clay on him a few minutes after the incident happened.

The results were incredible. Within two days, the injury had closed to approximately three inches. A cut, or a laceration heals like a zipper, from the inside out. With the clay, the healing time borders on unreal, relative to the amount of time conventional healing takes, especially if one gets the clay on quickly, while the wound is still fresh. You have to experience this phenomenon to believe it. This also applies to post-surgical wounds.

At last report, Jamie and Martha were doing fine. Betty decided to make a new life elsewhere.

Chapter 11

First Things First

Our deeds determine us, as much as we determine our deeds.

George Eliot

The summer of '87 came as a fierce reality check. When everyone said the area closed down, they weren't kidding. I remember days upon days when not a single car drove through Tecopa Hot Springs. Our area became a virtual ghost town physically and emotionally. The little community simply withdrew from the world. Like one of those small frogs in a dry creek bed, Tecopa Hot Springs instinctively dug in and patiently waited for the Snowbirds and the Season of Plenty to come again in the fall.

I can safely say that without the clay's possibilities seducing my imagination, I'd have already left, cut my losses, and resumed my career. But I was hooked. Obviously, the clay was potentially a great therapeutic service. With this tremendous prospect came a growing stack of unresolved circumstances and questions:

1. What must we create?

2. How do we manage the logistics of the clay?

3. How would the clay be prepared, handled, and cared for on a daily basis?

4. What other facilities must we design and build in order to take the clients through the entire process of this new service?

First, I needed to grasp the extent of what I didn't know. Because the clay occupied all my waking thoughts, there surfaced the vague scenario that the ripple effects could be powerful enough in the right setting to effectively counter the "Tecopa Hot Springs–Closed for the Summer" syndrome. Summer, or no summer, I couldn't let my interest in the clay distract me any longer from everything that needed my attention.

I enjoyed the metaphor describing what the old evangelist adhered to: "You have to get 'em into the tent before you can save em!" That particular adage–American as apple pie–seemed to hit the bulls-eye for much of what I immediately faced.

We needed to completely rebuild, remodel, and rethink everything on my property to somehow integrate it with what I was somehow going to create for the therapeutic clay.

I wrote myself notes, all kinds of notes, and this particular note stood three feet tall and 18 inches wide. I made an all-inclusive list in large script of what I needed to do, and in what order. I then ceremoniously attached the proclamation on a wall in the front room/office where everyone gathered every day.

To Whom It May Concern
The Situation
We Must Assume

1. For all practical purposes no one on Earth knows where Tecopa Hot Springs is located.

2. If by some remote chance they've heard about where we are then they've also been made aware that we're basically closed during the summer.

3. If our potential client has heard enough to know we're so close to Las Vegas, but we're closed in the Spring till Fall, then they also know that even in Season there are no other services to speak of, and those we would speak of are in sad shape.

Be It Known On The Plus Side We Have:

Excellent Hot Mineral Water. Quaint location. Good Weather, Free County Hot Baths, and cheap rates. Remember: This is what keeps the community hanging on!

The Summer of '87 Building Battle Plan:

Build or acquire new rentals. Remodel old ones. New outside restrooms. Rebuild swimming pool with new roof. New gift shop and office. Two new patios. Design sun/shade/wind structures. Design and build temporary clay pool. Outside showers. New hot tubs. Massive graveling. New parking lot.

The first time Curt saw the board he grinned and said, "Not too much, if you say it quick." Curt's dry sense of humor aside, he realized that to be even partially ready for what I wanted done by the fall season, and more importantly prepared for the crucial and decisive summer of '88, it would require that he get his crew started long before sun-up, then work hard and smart before the heat of the day hit. A tough summer was on us.

As Curt attacked his projects I too had a chore, I had to do some thorough research involving the use of clay. In two weeks I observed the services of every major spa in California. I quickly realized that since I wasn't interested in the conventional Spa feature of a cosmetic application of clay, I had to start from scratch to design multiple services and methods entirely original and functional for our purpose.

First, I would be using 100% pure therapeutic clay, and second, I was creating a setting specific for our environment, which was completely different from a standard cosmetic/ leisure-oriented high-end luxurious resort.

I realized that no one else out there was doing what I wanted to do, and no one shared my motivation. When I completed my tour of California spas, I had sketched out a fairly clear idea about how I wanted to construct my therapeutic Clay Center.

During my trip I saw many beautiful places, but none set up to handle a true all-around pure internal and external Therapeutic Clay experience. Those types of services fell outside their scope of business. Through this learning process came some important revelations concerning the type of clients I felt our operation would attract.

I bet our clients would appreciate that safe, inexpensive, active participation in their own well-being, stimulated by dramatic results, would provide the ultimate pay-off for their experience. It would cause them to spread the word and keep coming back. The idea was simple: we would not overly pamper. These people were coming to BE and to make themselves better.

After 2:00 a.m., I wearily pulled into my place. I had been gone for almost two weeks. I shut the engine off and laid my head back on the headrest. I had covered a lot of real estate, seen some elegant facilities, met some neat people, had a few real good times, and learned more than I expected. Exhausted and really too tired to sleep soundly, I toured the grounds to see what Curt had done. The man was unbelievable. He had accomplished far more that I ever imagined.

Invigorated and inspired to have this end of things in such able hands, I strolled about and relaxed without ever consciously thinking about where I was. I found myself up on the hill. I loved that hill. My thoughts took the form of sheer gratitude. To see what Curt had done, to be able to visualize what I was going to design for my Therapeutic Center, to know everything was going in the right direction was so very, very encouraging. "The play's the thing," and we were setting our stage.

I slept until almost noon, but heard no noise when I awoke. Unusual. There was always lots of noise because of construction and heavy equipment moving about. But not today. I finally woke up, showered, and looked outside to see why things were so quiet.

Curt had all the workers far in the back quietly cleaning and servicing our equipment.

He hadn't allowed anyone to come near where I was sleeping. That's the way Curt did things. I got some coffee and went out to see the workers. It was nice to be home. Curt had created a certain esprit de corps among his crew. They felt proud about what they were doing, and were glad for me to see their efforts.

We shook hands and Curt said, "Well, Cano, did you learn anything about what you don't know?"

I continued grinning and frowning, then said, "First, I have to understand the question. Ha! Yeah, yeah. I learned that we got a lot more here than we think we do."

He sat down on the tailgate of his old truck and asked, "How's that?"

"Well, in the first place, no one in California can do what we can do, mainly because they don't have what we've got to offer. They don't have the water, the location, the climate, or the clay! They don't have it, but even if they did, they don't want to do what we're gonna do!"

Curt said, "Sounds like you've learned some things and made up your mind."

"Yep. I have. What they call featuring a 'Clay Service' is a misnomer. They generally mix it with some stuff that's far from genuine. But it works for them. The customers have got nothing to compare it with. Understand though, most all of 'em are basically in the cosmetic business. People go there mainly just to relax, clean up, and get away. They whip it on 'em real good. Unbelievable prices!"

"Where'd you go?"

"I went up North above San Francisco, and then came down the coast, over to Palm Springs and down by San Diego. There's some mighty pretty spots, and darned expensive I might add, but high-end places or not, they can't do what we're gonna do."

Curt stood up and stretched. "You sound ready. I got the

notion you've got some ideas you want to kick around."

"As a matter of fact, I sure do. I've been thinking a lot about all the different things we got in front of us, but mostly about how to handle the clay and I'm real anxious for you to see what I've come up with for structures that can give us the option of shade or sun and a windbreak - all in one."

Curt paid close attention and said, "Oh? Shade and sun? That could be very important. I see you've been busy. It's good to have you home, Cano."

Chapter 12

It's A Keeper

Don't think! Thinking is the enemy of creativity. It's self-conscious, and anything self-conscious is lousy. You can't try to do things; you simply must do them. Ray Bradbury

I knew Curt would take a couple of hours to finish his work, so I used the time to review all my notes and sketches, preparing to acquaint my friend with the short and long term effort in front of us. That evening Curt and I spent seven hours discussing the project in detail. We went to Pahrump, Nevada, had a few drinks, talked through dinner, then returned, and continued to discuss our battle plan until late. During the evening I laid on the table a revised outline of exactly what we needed to create. I gave him priorities, and where I hoped we could be by fall, and pointed to the summer of 1988 as the date for total completion.

I kept the various designs for how to design and operate the clay pools, soaking pools and drying patios relatively simple. What I needed, but couldn't locate was a practical and functional method to give us the instant option of shade or sun, and could act as a windbreak when needed. I knew the problem; I just did not have a solution. While I didn't know exactly what I needed, I knew what I didn't want.

I knew I didn't want a structure with a solid roof or walls. A tent didn't quite work. I stayed with the premise that the structure must give the advantage of partial sun or shade as needed, and one should be able to quickly and easily assemble or disassemble the apparatus. In addition, it had to be strong enough to withstand a fierce desert wind, and yet be aesthetically pleasing.

I decided to utilize heavy-duty military parachutes. I would use the first ones, thirty feet in diameter, over the patios, and later over the clay and soaking pools. Ideally, ribbon chutes would give partial shade. These brightly colored chutes made of strips of tough nylon about two inches apart, are used by the Air Force as drag chutes for fighter jets. I knew the dry desert climate would preserve the fabric so the concept of a parachute for cover would theoretically work assuming the chute wasn't torn or deteriorating. My next problem came with creatively and adequately securing them, keeping them, here on Mother Earth.

For the first test structure, I planned to have Curt sink a series of eight thick iron pipes into two feet of concrete, spaced approximately twelve feet apart in a circle, thirty feet in diameter leaning outward and braced with two iron legs also set in cement. Then he joined the tops of these eight poles, each eight feet off the ground, with one continuous strand of 5,000-pound test steel cable. He then sunk a center brace, a telephone pole, into concrete, and it stood twenty feet high.

We would then drape the chute over the center pole, secure it, and hook it with quick release snaps to the steel cable running around the circumference of the structure. We could easily unhook the chute from the steel cable, and secure the whole thing in minutes. We could use ribbon or solid chutes as needed.

Late that evening after all the questions had been reviewed, new ideas considered, and all answered, Curt went first to the schematic diagram of the Sun/shade/wind structures, and studied them carefully. Then in an unusually quizzical fashion, he squinted and asked, "Cano, where did you ever see this?"

I just looked at him blankly for a second and said, "Curt, I didn't see it anywhere. Have you seen it before? I once saw part of a chute used as a screen, but this, I simply designed the structure to hold the chute in place, and make it easy to handle and all. What do you think?"

He kept examining my sketches. Suddenly, he took off his ball cap, rubbed his thinning hair, and mused, "By golly Cano! This'll work! And work well. Heck of an idea!" He laughed when he said, "The inspectors will have a time with these! Heh, heh, they sure 'nuf will. A hurricane or some of our storms might tear the chutes all up, but no kind of wind will ever harm the structure. I know some folks out here that would pay good money to have one like this!"

I loved his reaction. Combing his hair unconsciously with his fingers, and smiling broadly, he passed his judgment. "It'll work, Cano. This is a keeper. Customers will love it! When do I start on them?"

"Soon, my man, soon. But let's call it a night."

"Yeah, you're right. Time to shut 'er down. It's been a good one. See you in the morning."

Chapter 13

Little Al

The world is quickly bored by the recital of misfortune, and willingly avoids the sight of distress.   W. Somerset Maugham

After I'd been in Tecopa Hot Springs for a few months and had learned more about the healing clay, I spent the better part of each day talking to old-timers who had used it for years. I started to use the clay on everything possible. I began to compile a list of things that it worked on, and the results were remarkable. I couldn't get interested in anything that didn't have to do with my clay.

One day in Chino, California, a little girl had her knee sliced wide open, and very deep, on a piece of tin roof sitting on top of some junk. I was close-by when it happened. I saw her crying, the blood gushing, and the mother in a panic and nobody knowing what to do. The child's knee was cut to the bone.

I wrapped the knee with a towel, put the girl in my truck, and took both the girl and the mother to the emergency room of the local hospital. They cleaned the wound, stitched her up, gave her a prescription to prevent infection, and then handed the mother a bill that came damn close to what the girl's father earned in a month.

When I realized what I could have done if I'd only had my clay with me, I vowed never again to go anywhere, anytime without my clay. Never! The clay would have quickly stopped the bleeding, the possibility of any infection, and the pain. I also knew that the gelled clay, applied daily, would help the laceration to heal quickly, safely and without infection or scarring. A simple butterfly stitch would have sufficed.

Then there was Al.

I was on a mission to pass out some flyers in Pahrump, Nevada about our community's annual Fall Celebration Days. About a mile down a remote road, which existed only because it served as the entrance to a brothel of some fame, stood a strange bar that looked more like a small farmhouse. In front I saw a little broken down Toyota truck. It didn't look like it had been driven hard or abused, only that it had just gone a long way, and was tired. The truck was a friend to someone-an old, tired friend. The owner of this vehicle had a soft heart.

I wasn't too interested in the flyers I was distributing. We could put out a million of these things, and the same people would come who had been there the year before, and the year before that.

What I really wanted was a hot, buttered rum, or a straight-up double Bailey's with a cup of coffee. Funny, how you immediately like or dislike some places. This place was comfortable, warm, and someone had hit "Key Largo" on the jukebox, one of my all-time favorite songs. I love the line that says, *Here's looking at you kid, and all the things we did.*

When I walked in, this little bar had a total population of two. The bartender seriously looked like an ex-miner who couldn't stand the brutal work any longer, and who also enjoyed a little taste every now and then. I got the impression he would have worked for free just to get out of the house, and be able to have a straight shot at an appropriate moment, which came pretty often.

The other person sat passively preoccupied. The music stopped. He turned and glanced at me, and I saw a gentle, effeminate, and very sad soul. He rocked slightly on his stool, and tenderly held his left elbow. He seemed to be in pain. Then he stopped for a moment, stretched out his right hand, and softly flexed the fingers. He grimaced when he closed his fingers into a loose fist. He repeated this rocking motion, cradling his left arm, and then flexing the fingers of his right hand. A tear ran down his right cheek. He looked like a man with a heart that was about to break. I sat four stools to his right, and observed his obvious pain. The bartender asked, "What'll y'all have?"

I felt chilled and the guy on my left didn't exactly warm me up. "Hot buttery rum with a cinnamon stick?"

"Sorry, Mister can't fill that order."

"No problem, I'll have a double Bailey's in a cup of coffee."

"Man, that's two strikes on me. We're outta Baileys, but how about a Drambuie?"

I didn't really like that idea. "Fine, and a cup of coffee?"

He stuck up a big, gnarly forefinger and said, "Got it."

It was as if the little man was in a room by himself. I stole a glance or two at him. When the Drambuie and coffee arrived, I leaned over a bit and asked the bartender, "Is he okay? He looks pretty down."

The bartender turned his back to shield his voice a bit from the little guy, and whispered in a coarse, gravelly voice, "He's having a hell of a day." He motioned outside. "His story fits the weather. Get this: he's being evicted from the home he built! He just lost his job, but the reason he's so down, though, is because he had what many of us thought was the most beautiful dog in town, had him since he was a pup. He was killed last night by a bus on the highway. His name is Al. Nice little guy. Everyone likes him, and we all feel bad about it." He poured himself a shot, and said, "These damn buses drive like they own the road." He raised his glass, "To your health."

I looked at Al and recognized his fresh, raw grieving process. I took a sip of Drambuie. I don't like the stuff. It tastes like foul medicine. I chased the medicinal taste from my mouth with a swallow of nice, hot, black coffee. I began to warm up. Al saw me make a face when I sipped the Drambuie, like I was drinking raw lemon juice, and ever so slightly, he cracked a small grin.

I shook my head and asked him, "Would you like this Drambuie? I don't care much for it."

He didn't look like much of a drinker, but out of kindness, just to relieve me from looking at it in front of me, he replied, "Sure, I'd enjoy it. Thanks."

I leaned over and shoved it within his reach, and he seemed to brighten up a bit. He stretched his back and started rubbing his finger as if it were broken, or injured in some way.

I said, "Excuse me."

He turned toward me, still holding his finger.

"I can't help but notice, but what's wrong with your arm and finger?"

He tossed his head toward the outdoors, "It's the weather. I've got arthritis in my elbow and finger, and this sort of weather always makes it kick up. It hurts really bad."

The pain of losing his job, house, and dog wasn't helping matters any. I can't ever remember feeling so sorry for anyone. I mean, damn! How tough can it get?

"Could I look at your finger?"

His eyes told me that he appreciated my interest and concern for his plight.

I got up and walked to his side, "That looks like a splinter in the joint." It was the little finger of his right hand.

"It *feels* like a splinter too, but it's arthritis."

The knuckle glowed an angry red, as if a splinter had been driven deep into the tissue, and had festered there. I said, "It sure looks painful. I'm sorry that you're going through so much pain. And the arm?"

"Arthritis. But it's in the elbow. It's a more aching type of pain, but it hurts too." He sighed with an unconscious whimpering sound, as if he had no answers. Then he came back to me, "You're not from around here, are you?"

"No, I'm from Tecopa Hot Springs."

"Oh, I see. Well, Thanks for the drink, anyway." He shot me a polite half smile. The little guy sighed again, and solemnly broke off our conversation, then returned to the solitude of his grief.

"Excuse me again, but I think I can help you ease the pain in your fingers, and help with the elbow, if you'd allow me to try something."

Al looked askance at the bartender. The bartender had a shot and deliberately set the jigger down.

Al said, "Yeah? How?"

"Don't go anywhere, I'll be right back. I gotta get something out of my truck."

This is it! I thought to myself. This is the first time I get to use my clay on someone outside of my place! By then I always carried the clay in my truck, and had been doing so for several weeks. I would never again pass up the chance to put the clay on someone just because I didn't have it with me...

I brought in a small plastic tub of my clay, of the sort I gave away as samples, which were very popular. I called it "Seed Clay," and on the label it said:

SEED CLAY
Seed Money is Great
But, Seed Clay is
Beyond belief!!

I enjoyed sharing these samples, and we had given literally thousands away. Both of them could tell I was serious.

"Can I see your finger?"

It really looked like an infected splinter: red, swollen and painful. I held his hand, and applied the clay to his little finger.

"What do we do?"

"Nothing. We just take it easy, and allow it to dry."

"That's it?" He glanced at the bartender, at his finger, then back at me.

The bartender, looking incredulous said, "That's all?"

"Yep." I walked over to the jukebox, and selected "Key Largo" three times for my quarter.

After twenty minutes or so of small talk, Al reached over and picked up a glass of water.

The bartender had been observing Al fairly closely, and he barked, "Al! What are you doing?"

"Nothing. I'm not doing anything."

"The hell you're not! You picked up that glass with your right hand! You had your little finger wrapped around the glass!"

Al picked up the glass again with his right hand, then quickly set it down, and flexed his fingers. Little Al stood up, flexed his fingers, and stuttered, "My Lord! The pain's gone!" He looked at the ceiling, and shouted again, "My Lord! The pain's gone! Glory! Glory!" He began to sort of skip around the room, waving his arms.

The bartender had a new story to tell. "This is the damnedest, weirdest thing I've ever seen! Wait `till Helen hears about this!"

Al went on like one of those folks at a tent revival meeting.

Then a cold thought hit me: These two have set me up. They're putting me on. This is a show, an act and I went for it. I half-yelled, "Wait a minute! Hold on! Just wait a second!"

Al gave me a puzzled look

"Let me see the finger." I motioned to the bartender "Get me a small towel soaked in warm water, please."

Al looked at the bartender with big tears in his eyes. "It's gone, Howard. The pain is gone. It's a miracle, isn't it?"

"Damnedest thing I ever saw. Here's the towel you wanted."

I held Al's hand, and gently soaked the finger to remove all the clay. I put my glasses on to inspect the finger for myself. They weren't putting me on! The redness had completely disappeared. *Gone!* I rubbed his finger in a way that would have sent him through the roof twenty minutes before. Al laughed and cried at the same time. Almost hysterical, his emotions were almost over the edge, and I was doing pretty well, too.

I had never seen anything like it either. The inflammation had disappeared. I remember looking around the room at the tables and chairs, the jukebox, at Al, at Howard. I didn't ever want to forget the moment! In the next thirty minutes, we had Al's elbow in fine shape again, too.

Al said, "God does move in strange ways," and he began gently crying. Then between sobs said, "He took my beautiful dog away, and then brought me here to find relief for the terrible pain I've had for nine years! How do you figure that?"

Hell, by that time Al, Howard and I were all sniffling together. I decided we should all have a straight shot of strong whiskey, and listen one more time to "Key Largo."

⑃ ⑃ ⑃

Al used the clay on several more occasions, and he was one of the lucky ones whose arthritis never came back after treatment. Shortly thereafter, Al came to work for me as Head of Housekeeping at the Crystal Cross. Al was a true Clay Disciple and a dear friend.

Chapter 14

The Runaway Day

*Life loves to be taken by the lapel and told: "I'm with you kid.
Let's go."*   Maya Angelou

I thought, came up with ideas, and Curt built. Everything we
designed worked, and the folks coming by to indulge themselves in
our services left feeling great, and talking about us. The fact that
the customers had to step around our latest construction project
didn't bother them in the least. On the contrary, the effort they
made seemed to make them feel a part of the task.

We sailed through the fall of 1987 in great shape and actually
ahead of schedule.

In March of 1988 while Joyce conducted free Yoga classes for
some of the locals, I discussed Clay Therapy with a small group of
people from Las Vegas, while swimming.

Later, a man approached me and introduced himself, "Hi, I'm
Frank Crawley, and I'm curious. Do you ever listen to radio?"

"Ah, yes, when I'm driving, not here though. First, I don't
have time, and second, we don't get very good reception out here.
Why?"

He sat down on a bench and draped a towel around his neck.
Fat people look fatter when they sit down. Mr. Crawley,
considerably overweight, gave the impression he had given up

doing anything about the condition a long time ago. His hair was silver gray and he wore it long on the sides and past the collar in back. He had dark brown intelligent eyes, and a lot of hair all over his back.

He toweled off his hair and threw it over his head to form a hood and said, "Well, frankly, after listening to you discuss the uses of your clay, I kept thinking and wondering if you'd ever consider advertising on the radio."

"Oh, I see, do you sell advertising?"

"No, no. I'm a Chiropractor in Las Vegas."

"Ah, I got it! You're Mary Jo's husband. Crawley, is it? Sure, sure, glad to have you here."

He sipped an orange drink. "She's a big fan of yours, and got reason to be, the work you did on her feet and lower legs was amazing. I couldn't do anything with it. Edema is hard to treat."

"I appreciate it, Doc. I get a lot of credit for what the clay does. It makes us all look good, but the clay is the only healer around here."

I like to hear fat people laugh, which he was doing when he said, "Very well, I understand, but you're doing a heck of a job. Lots of folks are talking. Real interesting stuff. Took the swelling down exceptionally quick. Since she was out the first time, every other day or so does the trick."

"That's great to hear. I'll be glad when every chiropractor in the country knows how effective it is for a lot of things they treat."

Doc Crawley said, "I'd sure like to know more. I've been practicing for over 25 years and I agree, you could very well have something our profession could utilize in several ways."

"Thanks, Doc. I hope so, and you're right. I know of several uses that will surprise a lot of M.D.s and chiropractors as well, but why did you ask about the radio?"

He stood up and pulled on his shirt. "You know, it occurred to me when you were answering the questions, and I must say, you seem to really enjoy talking about the stuff, that if that conversation had been on the radio it would be very effective and generate a lot of interest. I was just curious." He picked up his pants and shook them out. "I listen to radio, talk radio. Big audience. I advertise. It's been real good."

He slipped his right pants leg on and as he attempted to put the left one on he tangled his foot, tripped and fell on to the cement floor directly on his left knee. The injury wasn't serious, but he did knock off a good chunk of skin and the wound bled pretty good.

"Damn it all. What have you got for a bandage?"

"Let me give you a hand, Doc."

He got back on the bench while still cursing the gods of fat.

I said, "I won't be sixty seconds, Doc. I got something better than just a bandage." I soon returned with a small amount of dry powered clay and a small sample tub of gelled clay.

I first covered the abrasion with the power, and waited for a minute or so, and proceeded to cover the whole area with the gelled clay. Then I waited for a moment because I knew what was coming.

"Mr. Graham, this is amazing! The stuff took the stinging away, almost instantly!"

I loved it. "Frank, call me Cano, please. Also, if you check, I think you'll find the bleeding has stopped too."

He fumbled around for his glasses, got them on, and examined his knee, "Well, I'll be go to hell. It stopped the bleeding and feels kind of like an anesthetic of some type."

"I know what you mean. Doc, leave that on until it all dries, then soak it off. By the way, where it sticks on the wound, just leave it alone and cover what's sticking with more of the gel."

He smiled at me. "You love this stuff, don't you? Heh, heh. Cano? Funny name. You don't worry about infections? I heard you talk about it but, even on this?"

"You won't either from now on. You'll see." I wrapped a piece of clean sheet around his knee so his pants wouldn't brush the clay off, "Okay, Doc, you're good to go."

Doc stood up, and moved the leg around to see that everything was in order. "Look Cano. I've got a golfing buddy who has a wife working at KDWN radio station in Las Vegas. She does commercials, Patricia Hill is her name, like I said they do talk radio, biggest in town, goes all over. If you're ever interested give me a call."

"Hey, thanks for the tip, Doc, but I've got a lot to do for awhile. I want to make sure our service is on line before I throw a lot of effort at marketing. We've still got a way to go. We'll make it, but we're not actually there yet."

As we left the dressing area, Doc said, "Mary Jo said you were really into this place. Now I believe it. Good luck!"

I shook his hand. "Thanks, Doc, and thanks for the radio tip. It would be great having a real pro doing commercials for us. I'll look at my options, and be in touch if I decide to go that way. Take care of yourself."

♳ ♳ ♳

A few days after my conversation with Doc Crawley, I was on my way home from Las Vegas in late afternoon. Tired from buying supplies all day long, I had a full load and just wanted to get home to the Crystal Cross. The last thing I needed was an accident, so I just held it on 55, and decided to find some good music and coast home without falling asleep at the wheel.

I dialed for the right sound, and finally landed on some station that had several guests talking about the benefits of massage therapy and other new age disciplines. Then they introduced a guest who discussed wheat grass. I wasn't interested in wheat grass or thinking about anything, so I flipped the dial, found some music, and settled back for the drive home. I could drive it in my sleep.

About that time my brain attacked me, and wondered, what the hell is wheat grass? And how can it possibly be interesting enough to be a major topic on a radio show? I couldn't shake the question so I turned the dial back to the wheat grass lady.

I began to listen carefully to the interview and to the people calling in. The announcer asked stimulating questions, and the wheat grass lady answered them in a reasonable fashion. The show took a commercial break, and I realized I had found KDWN in Las Vegas, Nevada.

This woman was establishing communication with how many thousands, tens of thousands, hundreds of thousands of people? After listening for half an hour, I was wide-awake and thinking. They were selling a ton of wheat grass. Wheat grass! I was totally re-energized. Commercials about The Crystal Cross would fit on that station. It could work.

I turned the volume up. They kept talking and I kept thinking. When I got to the Crystal Cross, Joyce was waiting with supper. "Hi, honey, you must be bushed with all you had to pick up. Why don't you take a shower and I'll set the table."

"Hi, Babe, Yeah, I am hungry, go ahead and set the table, but shower? No, I've got to make a phone call."

"Oh, honey, you've had a long day. Slow up. Take a shower. I've got a nice dinner here."

I kissed her cheek. "Thanks, honey. Okay, I'll take a shower, but I've got to make one quick call to Las Vegas." I grabbed the phone, kicked back in my recliner and dialed the number. "Hello, Mary Jo? This is Cano Graham at the Crystal Cross in Tecopa Hot Springs. Oh, fine, feeling great. Yes, please put him on. Hi, Doc, Yes, since you mentioned it. Set me up an appointment with KDWN. I'm ready!"

               C03   C03   C03

Early mornings, Curt and I did our best thinking and planning over coffee before the crew arrived.

"Curt, I'm thinking of advertising for the coming summer. Will we be ready, for sure? Can we go for it?"

"Just depends. We can be ready. The question is for what? How much has to be done?"

"Alright, here it is. I know we have a long way to go, but just for this summer, I need a particular blend on line."

"Okay, how many rooms?"

"No rooms, we don't need more rooms."

"I don't get it. Why not rooms?"

"I want to ask you something that has to do with an idea I got. It's my understanding that in Tecopa Hot Springs nobody's ever made any effort to make allowance for people who simply want to use their hot baths for a few hours. Why is that?"

"Easy enough. All the owners have hot baths, of course, but they're just for their customers. And naturally doing it this way made sense because the county has free men's and women's hot Baths, and a lot of folks enjoy 'em. The county baths aren't real attractive to many of the tourist though. The county doesn't keep them as they used to and they're getting old. But they work fine for the price of admission."

"Yeah, I see, they're free! The locals are used to 'em. It's a social thing, a habit; it's where they go, okay, but not for others. Here's what's on my mind Curt. I'm not concerned about them staying all night. I want to get 'em here for a few hours, so they can use what we offer and be back in Las Vegas by evening, feeling good and talking about us."

"You mean by the hour?"

"No, by the day. One charge for everything. Swimming pool, clay bath, hot tubs, everything we have for all day, like a theme park, and they can still get back home before dark."

"How much will you charge?"

"Oh, I don't know. Not much. I want to give a lot of people from Las Vegas a good taste of what we have, and send them home happy." I laughed, "Curt, I'd pay them, but I'll probably charge them , oh say, twenty dollars a piece for the entire day."

"That's a keeper Cano, but you could easily double the fee.

They'll love it. Why couldn't they bring a lunch with them and have a picnic under the patio chute?"

"Great idea, Curt." I smiled at the big guy. "That'll work! I want to create a buzz. Like the old preacher said, 'We got to get 'em into the tent before we can save 'em.'"

"What do you see we need to make it work?"

I shifted in my seat with excitement. "Okay, I'd like to have three new clay pools ready, different sizes. For the idea to work, we'll need a large area for them to dry the clay. We know that outside is great on most days, but we need a solarium for inside drying. Besides showering the clay off, I have an idea about a soaking pool, only about eighteen inches deep. I've got some sketches."

Curt furiously made notes. "If we don't run into any problems the swimming pool will be fixed in a couple of weeks, so that's out of the way. But you know, a situation that could turn into a real nuisance is the parking. We need to grade and gravel for parking."

"That's for sure. I was coming to that problem, and you know something else? We need to add to our dressing areas."

Curt looked over his notes. "We can get it all ready, but how you gonna tell the story to get 'em here? Most of 'em will think they're being invited to a picnic in a morgue called Tecopa."

"Exactly right. Commercials have got to explain the difference. You know the difference between a morgue and a dance hall? They both got people?"

He smiled at me. "I don't know, but I think you're gonna tell me."

"Yeah, well, one's got action and one don't. We're gonna create action. We're gonna get 'em up and moving in this direction and we'll take care of 'em when they get here and send 'em home wanting more!

"If you can do that, I'll get it built."

ଔ   ଔ   ଔ

I called Doc Crawley. He said, "I talked with Pat Hill yesterday, she was set to present a series of commercial ideas to you, but she started talking with one of the announcers, and things turned a different direction."

"Oh, what's up now?"

"Cano, do you remember a boy and his mother that were out to your place not too long ago? The boy had a bad case of acne. Name is Anthony Lane?"

"No, no I can't recall."

"The kids a whiz at playing the sax. You got to see him perform one night. His mother used to act."

"Oh, sure, Tony, Tony and his mother Beth!"

"Yes, that's them. Anyway, it's a small world. Turns out that Beth and Tony think you built the world. The clay you gave them cured the acne, but get this, Beth and Tony are the wife and son of Doc Lane the announcer at KDWN radio. Hell, he already knows you, and wants you to do a thirty minute spot on their Friday afternoon call-in show that deals in New-Age stuff!"

I was thrilled. "Doc that sounds like a winner!"

"All the way! This could be better than what I first discussed. Just talk to them, Cano. Tell the Clay Story like you told us that day in the pool."

ಛ   ಛ   ಛ

My nerves jangled as the show started. I kept thinking about how many people were listening. I didn't feel good about the way it went with the first few callers. I didn't feel close to them. Then I realized what was wrong. I wasn't really listening to the caller. I heard them, but as they spoke, I considered how to respond to thousands of people at once. I started carefully identifying with what each caller said, and proceeded to shut out all the rest of the audience and discuss clay therapy with just that individual. It was like we got to know each other. Older people who knew about

Clay Therapy started calling. A kindred spirit between the Clay and the audience seemed to grow, and I recognized a tangible enthusiasm. Everything was going very well, but I was waiting for a certain question. It came when a woman called about the room rates for herself and her two children.

"Do you intend to spend the night?" I asked.

"Well, I want to come out and spend some time, so I need a room."

Ma'am, you don't need to spend the night unless you want to. We have day rates. You can come out, spend all day if you wish, swimming, Clay pools, hot baths, take a walk, whatever, and bring a picnic lunch, and come back home at night."

"What are the day rates? I have two children."

"How old are they?"

"My children are seven and ten, both boys."

"The cost is twenty dollars."

"Oh, that's twenty dollars apiece?"

"No, ma'am, that's twenty dollars for you. Children under twelve are free."

I could've kissed her when she said, "Good heavens, are you open tomorrow?"

"We sure are."

"This is the best thing that has happened to me since I won a jackpot at the Stardust. Thanks, see you tomorrow."

I said, "Bye, see ya then."

Then came the splash of cold water. An older gentleman called in, and said that he for one didn't believe for a second that our clay would do what I said for his wife's arthritis, and his feet, and he wasn't coming to throw away good money.

"Who am I talking to?" I asked.

The old fellow said, "This here's Paul Douglas, we just moved down here from Reno."

"Well, Mr. Douglas, do you know where Tecopa Hot Springs is located?"

"No, in fact the Missus is trying to find it on the map. You say it's west of Vegas about 80 miles? Oh, she says she found it."

"Fine, Mr. Douglas. I want you to understand something. Now this isn't just for you and Mrs. Douglas. This is for everyone, everyday. This is how we operate. When you come to the Crystal Cross Therapeutic Center, and you have a problem, like your feet or Mrs. Douglas' arthritis, if you don't feel that the Clay works to your satisfaction, or if you don't feel as good as you think you should, then you don't pay. That's it. If our clay doesn't work, then you don't pay!"

"Well I'll be darned." I suppose he was talking to his wife who was listening on her radio. We could hear him say, "Jinny, did you hear that?"

"I hope I meet you, Mr. Douglas."

"You will, you will, and you'll meet Jinny too!"

The station took a commercial break. Doc Lane said, "If it doesn't work they don't pay? Hey Cano! You're ready to back that up?"

"Oh, yeah, I'll back it up all day everyday

"Man, you're creating some interest today."

"Great, I was just wondering, I've already gone over the half hour, how long does this go on?"

Doc and the engineer started laughing and pointed at the bank of buttons. "See all those buttons all lit up?"

"Yes, it looks good to me."

The engineer said, "Ha, you *should* feel good. People are holding and waiting to talk to you. Some are calling long distance. If you like the response, imagine how we feel? This is what we call a hit. The sponsors love it; the station loves it; the callers love it. You're not going anywhere. Some call this a Runaway Day."

Runaway Day! After two hours the station brought the show to a close, and the telephones were still blinking. They invited me back for another show. Doc Crawley and Mary Jo were at the station when we finished the show, and we celebrated like an

136

opening night party.

Although alone, I managed to fully enjoy the drive back to the Cross. I was just sailing along, laughing and carrying on. When I got back, Joyce, Ruthie, Beulah, Mori, Art, Luella, Sylvia and Curt were all waiting for me and we partied till late. Joyce had taped the entire two hours of the show, and we had a great time replaying some of the important calls.

A knock on the door came just after Curt got to work on Saturday morning, and that means early! The first words I heard gave his identity away.

A little old guy said, "Where's this man Cano Graham? He said that we don't pay if the Clay don't work!"

I opened the screen door. "Come in Mr. Douglas."   Then I looked past him and said, "Jinny, I'm sure glad you're here. You folks care for some coffee? I know you had to have started early this morning."

Mr. Douglas said, "Oh that would hit the spot. Yes, yes, we like to get an early start."

I smiled and offered the couch. "Make yourselves comfortable."

It was the start of the summer of 1988 and the snowbirds were gone. We were ready, and they were coming. Paul and Jinny Douglas were the first of many that weekend. The word about us spread around Las Vegas and they kept coming and left feeling better than when they arrived. We had a Runaway on our hands.

Chapter 15

The Sting

People are inexterminable–like flies and bed bugs. There will always be some that survive in cracks and crevices- that's us.

Robert Frost

I had just returned from Denver, Colorado and was anxious to catch up on all the new developments in my absence. We were in the process of building the new Therapeutic Clay pools on a larger scale than anywhere else. I found this a very exciting time.

While at dinner in Denver, I had invited several people to come in a few months to Tecopa Hot Springs to enjoy the hot mineral water, healing clay, and the great weather. We kept ourselves busy with new constructions and were, at present, discouraging customers because the timing was bad.

Of all the people in Denver, the one man who I frankly didn't care to see, and especially hear again, was an obnoxious loudmouth who delighted in sick, off-color jokes in a mixed crowd of people he didn't know. I figured this guy for a certifiable creep. The sad part of this little story was that he was now on the phone telling me that he had just rented a motor home and was on his way for the clay!

I really didn't want him near me, certainly not around my other guests. But nonetheless, a few days later he appeared along with some bizarre stories of his trip and an even more bizarre blonde girlfriend who definitely belonged with him. She laughed at every crude remark. By the end of the second day, everyone who met him shook their heads and began avoiding him. To even consider that they'd stay for two weeks was obscene. At the darkest hour, the Lord provided a small miracle of sorts.

I had just returned from Las Vegas when the repulsive creature came running toward my truck yelling, "Liz has been bitten by a scorpion. Where's the closest doctor?"

"One thing at a time. First, she wasn't bitten, she was stung. And second, the closest doctor is in Las Vegas, eighty miles away. How bad is it?" I sensed the chance of a lifetime, to kill two birds with one shot. I tried not to sound overly excited. "Where is she?"

I had heard about scorpion stings before and about the effectiveness of the Therapeutic Clay in stopping a bad insect sting of any kind, but I had heard all the scorpion stories second hand. I had heard that if the Clay was put on a scorpion sting quickly, within a minute or so, that it would never develop the normal symptoms of swelling and pain. I don't like to see anyone in pain, but if it had to happen, I felt very lucky to see one first hand. The cats at the place snuffed the scorpions as fast as they found them, so this was a true blessing for me. I also sensed other benefits, but I wasn't sure what they might be. For now, I grew excited by the wonderful news.

I've always been lucky. She had been stung several hours earlier when she stepped barefoot out of the motor home. I'd be less than candid if I didn't admit that on some level, in some small way, I enjoyed Al's panic. He reminded me of what I thought Al Capone would have been like.

Thrashing his arms in anguish he said, "We're just getting used to this place, the desert and all, and then this has to happen!" We had almost reached the motor home. He was halfway running and asked, "Does this happen often?"

"Very rarely," I said. "I hope she doesn't lose her leg."

"Lose the leg!" he screamed. His terror and panic were beautiful to behold. I know I'll probably do time in purgatory for that enjoyment, but oh, what the hell. I put my finger over my mouth and said, "Shhhhush!"

He blinked and in a private sort of whisper said, "She might lose her leg? Christ!"

I cautioned him again. "Shhhhush," This was drama. "She might hear you and could die of shock in her condition. You know what I mean?"

"Oh, yeah," he said, now very aware and sympathetic.

I had the distinct impression that once and for all I could housebreak this creep and his lady creep.

The leg presented a lovely sight. Up to the knee it looked like the stub of an old, weathered fence post. It was perfect. I decide to push it just a little bit more. I was inspired.

"Oh, my God!" I yelled. "It's about to blow up!"

Al was in another zone. "Blow up?" he asked incredulously.

As I said, I was inspired. Brando would have been proud. I told him, "In some rare cases, a Death Valley type of scorpion sting would just blow with blood and stuff going off in all directions and the really bad part was that a heart attack would usually follow."

I was very clinical with my delivery. What a moment! She was near mute and he was limp.

"We should never have come. She could die. Oh, God! Help me."

I felt it was time to bring them back. I said, "I'm so sorry. I wish I could make you both feel better. By the way, did you hear this joke about the traveling salesman and farmer's daughter?"

He erupted. "What the hell are you talking about? This is no time for a joke!"

I said, "Oh no? I just thought I'd try to make you both feel better. Sorry." I kept my cool. This was just too good. I frowned and became very pensive. "Why didn't you put this clay on it when

140

you were first stung?"

"Clay?" she said.

"Yes." I pointed to some clay on their table. This cookie jar of gelled clay would have stopped the scorpion sting from ever swelling in the first place, but not unless you take it out of the jar and apply it all over the affected area. May I?"

"May you what?" she asked.

"The clay dear, the clay. We need to cover your entire lower leg good and thick in order to stop the pain and reduce the swelling."

"You mean the clay will stop..."

"Yes, if it's not too late."

They both exclaimed, "Too late!"

As I applied the clay, I told them how lucky they'd been, and that I was sorry to tell them that it wasn't a good idea to stay any longer because another sting could be the end. For the first time they grew silent, and in complete agreement suggested that they should leave the next morning.

At the time, a dermatologist named Dr. A. C. Howard was a guest. I stopped by the room he shared with his wife and mother and asked the doctor if he cared to examine a scorpion sting. I explained that the leg was badly swollen, that I had covered it up to the knee with thick clay and had instructed the couple to let it dry completely and then to soak it off and reapply. We filled our coffee cups and started over to my victim's motor home. Before we got within twenty feet of the door it flew open, and there in all his splendor stood good ole' Al in his underwear. Why do fat guys' underwear always look like it needs changing? He was in fine form, and seemed so happy to have survived the night.

"I can't believe it!!" he wailed. "Too much, man. Liz! Get out here!" he blubbered. "I wish we didn't have to leave, but like you said, one more sting and it could be curtains." He clearly wanted to appear heroic when he added, "Besides, Liz isn't too crazy about the desert. Liz, get out here!"

No sooner said than done. There she stood, like Miss America stepping down the stairs. She made her debut in a short bathrobe.

"Can you believe it?" Al said.

I just hoped this wouldn't get too tacky. I said, "Doc, which leg was stung? Can you tell?"

Al said, "Are you a real doctor? Yeah? Ha. You won't believe this. She was near death last night."

The doc glanced at me with a puzzled look. I shrugged.

Dr. Howard picked up quick and said, "Let me look at this. Well!"

Liz then kicked her leg out from her robe like Marilyn Monroe giving the boys a thrill, then the other one. The doc looked at me. The girl did have nice legs. Only when she opened her mouth everything fell apart.

The doc laughed lightly and said, "Okay, I give up. Which leg was it? Was it really bad?"

I smiled broadly for a couple of reasons. One was because the stingees were packing and the other was because I wasn't sure which was more effective, the scorpion's sting or mine. The doc was smiling too. He got it loud and clear.

In his most aloof medical manner, the doc said to them, "You folks sure are lucky. Lucky indeed."

This was better than crunchy peanut butter in oatmeal. "By the way, Al, stop by the office before you head out. I've got a bucket of clay for you to use when you get home. It's on the house."

He said, "Thanks a lot, Cano."

Okay, so I recognized a certain sort of humanity about this guy, the byproduct of a recent near-death experience.

"Thanks so much." And then he said what seemed to be a strange thing coming from him, "You know, the Lord sure does move in mysterious ways."

"Yep," I said. "She sure duz."

142

Chapter 16

Bob and Helen

Fate leads the willing, and drags along the reluctant.   Seneca

At about 10:00 p.m. on April 14, 1988, the rain came down like cats and dogs and the wind blew like a gale. The buzzer in the office rang. I threw my robe on, flipped on some lights and opened the door. "May I help you?"

This worried soul looked at me and said, "Yes, yes I need a room, and is there a Doctor around here?"

"I can help you with a room, but there isn't a Doctor. The closest would be in Pahrump, Nevada, about twenty-five minutes away. What's the problem?"

"We're from Bishop on our way to Las Vegas. My wife started getting sick just after we ate in Lone Pine. She's getting sicker by the minute. We think she might have food poisoning. I ate different than she did. I'm not sick. I'm afraid to drive on to Las Vegas. Maybe I should go to where you said, Pahrump?"

Food poisoning? Great! I'd seen a lot of different problems lately, but I hadn't yet had the chance to put my clay into an active, in-progress food poisoning case. And I had one sitting out there in the car! I didn't want them to get away. "Did you come through any high water?"

He was thinking. He rubbed his stomach a little bit, and let out a sigh of exhaustion, and a long deep sigh. "No. No high water.

143

This is flash flood country, isn't it? Hmmm. No Doctor around, huh?"

"Nope. Do you know where you are?"

"Tecopa Hot Springs?"

"Right, but do you know the name of my place? Do you know what we do here?"

"No, I don't know. I just saw the sign. A center of some kind? It's raining hard. I just followed the arrow."

The wind was picking up. She started leaning on the horn. "Oh-man!" He shook his head. This man was between a very big rock and a hard place.

"You chose the right place. This is the Crystal Cross Therapeutic Clay Center."

"Is it?" he replied. "You helped a friend of mine, a highway patrolman from Death Valley, with an abscessed tooth. Do you remember him? Collins, Richard Collins?"

"Yeah, I know Dick. In fact he's working this area now."

"So this is the Clay place? I'll be darned. Are you Cano?"

"Yep, I sure am." As we shook hands the horn started blaring again. The wind started howling too, big time. "I think you should stay here. I've got a nice room for you and more importantly, I've definitely got something for you wife. Fill out the card and pull your car around to number two. By the way, what's the name?"

He looked a little relieved. "Akins. Bob and Helen Akins."

Some sick is worse than other sick, and this lady was sick to the max. She was exhausted. I don't like to see people sick, but I was thrilled to have such a good case of food poisoning to work on. In this case, it was a cream soup that I had to thank. I thought she should start with a third of a cup. She drank some more and started to relax.

"Why don't you try to sleep?" I suggested. "I'll wake you in an hour or so and we can get some more in your system."

Bob pulled at his stomach and twisted up his face a bit, as if he'd done that same move a million times. "Bob, would you care for some Bailey's Irish Cream?"

"Helen, did you hear that?" he turned to his wife, "This man's got some Bailey's!"

She said, "Later…too much…whew, I think I feel better. Good night, boys."

Yahoo! I'd just seen my lady kick the ass of a bad case of food poisoning.

Helen slept and we drank Bailey's and talked. After a while, we realized the rain and the wind had stopped. Bob and I stepped out into a brilliant, diamond-filled sky. At Tecopa Hot Springs, we have no lights to speak of, so just after a fast moving desert storm it was a spectacular night. No air is quite as tasty as the desert air after such a cleansing as ours had just experienced. We didn't speak for a while.

"Hell of a night," I finally said.

"Yeah. Some coincidence, huh? Us pulling in here and all. Richard will flip."

"You want to take a short walk? The road is gravel. It's not muddy. In fact, we could go up on the hill. I can show you a heck of a sight. Helen is resting fine and we won't be gone but twenty minutes or so."

"Sounds great! I'd enjoy that."

As we strolled up the hill, Bob looked around and said, "Whoa, this is nice. Very nice! What a night! I want to show Helen this."

His remark brought me back.

"Glad you like it, but let's get back and check on Helen. I've got to be in L.A. by 9:00 a.m., so I need to turn in pretty quick. I have a very special breakfast date."

We found Helen sleeping like a baby. She had gotten up and put her nightgown on. She had poured herself a glass of clay water and had another one on the nightstand. It doesn't get any better than this!

"How long are you going to stay in Las Vegas?" I was hoping

145

they'd stay.

"We thought we'd be there for a long weekend. I've got an extra day off. We're just gonna take it easy, see some shows, play a little golf. Kick back, you know?"

Helen mumbled, "We're not going anywhere. This is it. We're not leaving." She had overhead us. There was a certain pleading in her request.

Bob said, "Have you got a room for us over the weekend?"

"I'll find one."

"Well that's a winner." Helen didn't even open her eyes. She said, "Thanks Bobby." She turned over towards us, woke up a bit and reached for her clay water. "Honey, this stuff is unbelievable. I mean, what's it been? Two hours? I heard you two talking. This is the place Richard Collins was talking about, isn't it? I've been drinking clay, haven't I?"

"You sure have! Do you really feel that good? No Vegas?"

"We can play right here, Dear." Helen was tired.

"Folks, I've got to get some shut-eye. Big day tomorrow."

They both started to talk at the same time. "Thanks so much."

I stopped them. "You'll never know how much I've enjoyed the last two-and-a-half hours. It's been a real pleasure, one I'll never forget."

Bob was kicking off his shoes. He reached into his shaving kit and pulled out a prescription bottle.

"What's that for?" I had to ask.

"Ulcers. Had 'em for six years. This is Tagamet."

After he said that, he just stood there and I just stood there. None of us said anything for a few seconds, but we were all thinking the same thing. Me, because I'd had some experience with ulcers and clay, and them because they were spellbound "Bob, you've been taking Tagament for six years?"

"Yes," he replied, sitting down.

Then Helen spoke up, "He's been through hell with 'em, too!" They just stared at each other. She shouted out, "Oh my God! Is it possible?"

"I want to tell you both something. This was my first chance to get a shot at a real good food poisoning case. I'm happy for all of us, but ulcers? I've had some dealings with ulcers. I don't know for sure how, I don't know why, but I do know that you just might have taken your last Tagament. Are you hurting now? I mean right now?"

"You damn right well better know that I'm hurting right now!"

"Good!" I said, already pouring out a glass of clay water for him. "Drink this now, and if you get up to pee, then drink another. I'm going to be gone in the morning, but this is the schedule. First thing in the morning and last thing at night, for two weeks or so, also have a glass or two during the day. You can't go wrong. Just put the powdered clay into water and swish it around, but don't let any metal touch the clay. No metal spoons or pitchers, okay?"

He drank it down and looked at her. "There's no taste to it. Sort of like a slight dusty taste?"

"All right, I'm gone folks. Tomorrow, do yourselves a full body clay bath along with the hot baths. I'll leave a note with Joyce. She'll fix you up. You'll love it! See ya!"

At 5:00 a.m. as I pulled out for L.A., Bob came running out of his room. "Hey, Cano, hold up, man! It's gone! I've had no pain at all. I know it's kind of early, but I feel great. I'll let you know how it goes."

He stood in his pajamas and his robe going on and on about how Helen was feeling. It had been a memorable six-and-a-half-hours. All of this and I was on my way driving through a refreshing desert to see the person I loved most on this earth, my mother. I couldn't wait to tell her about Bob and Helen. She loved to hear the latest news about our clay. She was one of the first Clay Disciples. Bob and Helen Atkins were the latest. I was to meet them again, too.

They had a wonderful weekend. Helen felt brand new the next

day and I got a letter from Bob three months later. I hung it in my office. Bob never took another Tagament, or anything else for an ulcer. The ulcer was gone. He took his clay regularly though, and he spread the word about it in lots of interesting places.

Chapter 17

Johnny Diamond

Even imperfection itself may have its ideal or perfect state.

Thomas De Quincey

Johnny was a Damon Runyon character incarnate. When the great street hustlers get together in heaven to rap, sooner or later, they'll get around to Johnny Solomon.

Johnny, a Jewish boy from Philly, found himself in North Carolina during the first part of World War II. His story really started when he began to hustle the sailors late into every night. Johnny had more tricks than Harry Houdini. He could do it all. His real name was Johnny Solomon, but many called him Johnny Midnight because he seldom left home until late, hitting the streets around midnight.

This little man married Lucia Bryant, one of the most beautiful, tall, willowy blondes anyone had ever seen. He could do three things better than anyone on the street, no matter where the street was. He could fight like a cornered wolverine; he knew diamonds like Harry Winston; and he could shoot pool on the level of Minnesota Fats.

Anything he tackled, he did better than anyone around, but he really loved to dance. He was constant motion on the dance floor. People swore he could levitate. His feet were a blur, and he cleared the floor nightly. He grew into a legend in Southern California. He never drank alcohol because he didn't want anyone to have an edge. He just chain-smoked and thought about his next hustle.

Johnny's ex-wife, Lucia, the tall blonde from North Carolina, was a close friend of mine. She knew first hand of my interest in clay, and one day in October 1989, she said, "Cano, Johnny's got a problem and I was wondering if..."

"About what? What's the problem?" She had confided in me that his health wasn't too good, but I didn't know too much beyond that.

I'd never met Johnny, but I'd heard a lot of stories. I knew he had long ago stopped fighting, and his pool playing days, along with the dancing, came to a halt one night when something happened. Nobody seems to know exactly what it was, but he simply said, "No more. I'll never dance or play pool again."

I imagine it was because he was the best, not just good, but the best. If he couldn't be the best, he wouldn't do it.

But, now he had a problem that he couldn't think his way out of. He'd had by-pass heart surgery, and the leg they'd stripped the veins out of just wouldn't heal. His doctors tried and tried, but nothing they did helped to heal his leg. A nurse regularly went to his home to change the dressing and apply medication. He ate pills like candy. But nothing helped.

Lucia finally asked me, "Would you talk to him?"

"Sure Lucia. I'll be more than glad to talk to him. I'd really like to see the problem though." After all the incredible stories I'd heard about this man, I just had to meet him.

His home was like walking into a dark, smoky saloon.

"So you're Cano, huh?" He sat at the kitchen table with a pot of coffee, and an ashtray full to the brim with smelly cigarette butts. "Coffee?"

I nodded. "How's it going, Johnny?"

As I began to ask questions, I visualized young Johnny Diamond playing pool in the best rooms in the country,

150

immaculately dressed, then clearing the dance floor with his blazing athletic moves. And he always had a little velvet sack of quality diamonds that he'd hustle later that night. God help the gang of toughs who were jealous, and wanted to take him down! Their asses were grass, and he was a power lawn mower.

He answered, "How am I doing? I got problems, pal!" He pulled his leg out from under the table to show me a gruesome sight about four inches above the ankle. "It just won't heal. The doc says we can't wait any longer. Says I'm close to having serious problems. Gangrene is what he's afraid of." He gently pulled back the covering, exposing the infection, which looked like a rotten boiled egg that had been smashed. I noticed a certain fragrance, too. Johnny hated pain. A small situation was a big problem to him. He was behind the eight ball, big time.

I asked, "How long has your leg been like this?"

He looked embarrassed. "Too long. Day after tomorrow they're going to do a skin graft."

"Are you scheduled for surgery?"

Lucia said, "He hates hospitals."

A kaleidoscope of his life passed before me again. I thought this life is a quick trip. "When does the nurse come again?" I didn't want her to interrupt my plan.

He said, "Tomorrow afternoon."

"Okay, Johnny, here it is straight out. Lucia has told you that I've had a lot of experience healing with clay right?"

"Yeah, come on, man. Clay?"

"It's a special type, okay?"

"Really?" He lit another cigarette from the butt of the one that still burned in the ashtray.

He glanced at Lucia and gave her a shrug of acceptance. I sure liked him. He needed me, and I was 100% convinced my clay would do the job. "Here's the deal, Johnny. Where's your antibiotics?"

He got them from the windowsill.

"You've got to stop taking 'em. The clay will suck 'em up getting at the infection anyway, so trust me, or rather trust the clay. You do what I show you two times today, and three times tomorrow, then if there isn't a very noticeable change by tomorrow afternoon, go ahead and have the skin graft done. If you see it obviously working then continue to follow the routine.

"Right now I'm going to apply a thick layer of clay, maybe a quarter-inch thick, and four inches in diameter. Leave it uncovered, then just kick back and let it dry. It'll take more than an hour, maybe two, but you can tell when it's dry. Then, use a warm towel, and soak off the remaining clay. Most of it will fall off, but the very center, where it's draining, the clay will tend to stick to it. Don't sweat it. Just let it stay, and cover the whole area again, then you repeat the whole routine. Got it?"

He nodded. I had his attention.

Also, I want you to drink a glass of clay water first thing in the morning, and again at night. On second thought, drink some throughout the day too. You're under a lot of stress. This will help."

"Cano, I've got a problem. What if the nurse catches me with the clay on my leg?"

I smiled a bit, "How long have you known her?"

"Quite a while. She's been coming here for some time. She's more worried than some of the doctors. At least, it seems that way … I don't know what she'd do. She's real fussy."

I loved this guy. Here he was with a leg that looked like an abstract painting, and he was concerned about a fussy nurse. I said, "She'll be here tomorrow?"

"Yeah, in the afternoon."

"Okay, we'll do it two times today. Then you apply one treatment again tomorrow morning, and have another one on and almost dry when she gets here."

"She'll flip."

"Johnny, when she sees the infected area tomorrow afternoon, if there's not a marked improvement, then get ready for a skin graft. By the way, where are they taking the skin from?"

He squirmed a little, "I'd rather not say."

"Okay, let's do it! Get me a warm towel please, Lucia."

I soaked the infected area, and rinsed out the center where it was suppurating. The skin was discolored, and very tight from swelling. I poured some dry, powdered clay directly into, and on top of the abscess. Then, I covered the whole area with a four-inch square of gelled clay, about one-quarter inch thick, and left it uncovered.

"Johnny, it's been great. I enjoyed your party, but we've got to go. We'll give you a call tonight. If we leave now, maybe we can beat some of the traffic. Take care of yourself, and remember, thoughts are prayers, and you'll be in our thoughts."

The air was fresh outside, but then any air would be fresh compared to the nicotine fog inside Johnny's kitchen. We stopped in Pasadena and had dinner. Lucia told me stories of Johnny's escapades. His life sounded like a miniseries, but I was more concerned about the ending.

When we walked into Lucia's home, two hours had passed since leaving Johnny's place. The telephone was ringing and Lucia answered it.

"Hello. Hi, Johnny. What do you mean where have we been? We ate dinner and drove home. What's wrong? What's unbelievable? Johnny, slow down. Yes, Cano is here. Yes, Cano is here-just a second." She motioned to me, "It's Johnny, and he wants to talk to you."

"Hey, Johnny, what's up?"

"Cano, I love ya, man. I can already tell it's working. I can feel it! Hell, I can see it. Hold a minute. I'm soaking it now. I can't believe this is my leg! These things happen to other people-like in the *National Enquirer*. Do you read the *Enquirer*?"

"No, I don't read the *Enquirer*, but describe the way it looks."

"It's not just how it looks, it's how it feels. I can literally feel it pulling the infection out. The swelling started to come down real quick. Man, it works! Do you want a partner? I can sell a ton of this stuff. I love it! Why isn't this stuff sold all over the world?"

I said, "Whoa, hold on, pal. First things first. Johnny, we're so happy for you, really, but take it easy!"

Johnny never needed the skin graft. His nurse showed up at the usual time the next day, and commented as she inspected the infected leg. "Never in thirty years of treating various infections have I ever seen anything like this!"

She immediately started treating her husband, who was suffering terribly with a rectal fistula, and his problem was solved. Johnny's leg healed quickly. In thirty days the new skin was pink, and healthy. He never took another antibiotic. The wonders of Mother Earth and her favorite daughter, handled the job just fine. Thank you.

Johnny was still living in the San Fernando Valley in Southern California when I last spoke to him. He still drank coffee, and smoked those damn cigarettes, while thinking about his next move.

His leg and heart have long since healed.

Chapter 18

Everybody Wins

The men who come on stage at one period are all found to be related to each other. Certain ideas are in the air.

Ralph Waldo Emerson

Few things in this life work out as well as we intend, but the Crystal Cross was an exception. I came to believe that if we had been only 20 miles out of Las Vegas, the whole idea wouldn't have worked. Las Vegas locals have a burning desire to get out of town. Tourists wanted to see the desert. And everyone wants a "destination." I started noticing rental cars and began to wonder how they had found us.

Finally, out of curiosity, I asked a couple, "How did you hear about us?"

The man said, "Where we rented the car. I told the fellow we wanted to see some things, not Boulder Dam because we had been there before. Anyway, he told us about this place. He said it was very un-Las Vegas." I laughed at that funny, although accurate description, said, "Thanks, enjoy the clay."

I went directly to the phone to call the car rental company that was directing customers our way. After getting the owner on the line and accepting his kudos for what we were creating, I said, "We sure appreciate your interest."

He said, "Our interest started the first day we heard you on that radio show. We listen while we work. As soon as you mentioned Tecopa Hot Springs, our salesmen examined a map and determined that the drive out and back was 150 miles. That's less than an hour and a half each way. Mr. Graham that's just a pleasant drive for a tourist, but it's a *trip* in our language. You must understand that the average rental in Las Vegas travels approximately seven miles." Then he started laughing, "You know what we call your place? How we describe the Crystal Cross?"

"No, I can't wait to hear a salesman's definition."

"Oh, you won't mind, it's catchy. We call it Primitive Elegance."

"Hey, I like that term. By the way, it's on the house for your employees. Just let us know who they are. We certainly appreciate the business. Keep those cars coming. I'll stop and meet you the next time I'm in town."

I got off the phone thinking a good deal is where everybody wins!

The Widgets Are Loose

In a full heart there is room for everything ,and in an empty heart there is room for nothing.

Antonio Porchia

Widgets are strange little things. No one has ever seen a widget. They have no shape or substance. They pop up from nowhere, mess around, and just as quickly fade into the nothingness from which they sprang. They aren't funny, and are sometimes even cruel.

When they come in bunches, they can drastically alter a perfectly happy life. They seem to come in cycles, monthly cycles, in fact. Almost every month, for some women, the widgets attack like a swarm of locust. Many times, the husband or another

156

member of the family will notice them first. In despair, he will utter the ominous phrase, "Oh, God, no! The Widgets are loose!"

Robin, a lovely, thoughtful, professional 45-year old, Susan, her mother in law, and Robin's 15-year-old son Larry, Jr. had decided to again flee Las Vegas for a long weekend in Tecopa Hot Springs. Robin's husband, a veteran Captain on the Las Vegas Fire Department, had decided not to come with them.

I thought at first, besides a get-a-way weekend, they came to treat Susan's arthritic hands and feet, and Larry Jr.'s recurring acne problem. Robin, a top-flight legal secretary, loved the hot baths. I'd never seen her any other way than completely delightful.

Susan had enjoyed her life as a housewife. She raised her family, did her daily work with a wonderful attitude, was devoted to her husband and children, and was the rock of her family. She had lost her first husband thirty years previously in a boating accident.

All boy, Larry, Jr. loved the clay pits, and jumped at the chance to help clean and refill the bigger ones. He was having a great time with the workers, when I realized that I hadn't seen his mother.

"Hey, Larry, Did your mom go to town? I haven't seen her today."

"Naw, Mr. Graham, she hasn't been out of her room yet. The widgets are loose!"

"Say what? The what's are loose?"

Larry, Jr. wiped the powdered clay off his face as he spoke, but he wasn't accomplishing anything except smearing it, which caused him to look like a clown.

He finally gave up the task, threw his hands out and said in a very matter of fact voice, "The widgets are loose. That's what my Dad call's 'em. When Mom doesn't feel good, Dad says, 'The widgets are loose.'"

I wondered what the hell the kid was talking about.

I turned around to see who was behind me, and there stood

Joyce with Susan.

Susan and Joyce had been talking on the beautiful, parachute-covered patio over coffee when Larry and I had our conversation about the widgets.

Joyce said, "Cano, Susan would like to discuss something with you. How about over lunch at the Miner's Diner?"

Susan smiled. "I'm buying."

"Hey! I can't pass up a free meal, just give me a minute to clean up."

We arrived at the Miner's Diner, sat down and ordered our food. I waited expectantly for Susan to open the conversation.

"Thanks for taking the time. I wanted this to be private," she said.

"No problem Susan. If it's important to you, it's important to us."

"I've discussed this with Joyce and she feels the situation would be important for you. This is about Robin."

"I didn't see her today. What's wrong? What are the widgets?"

Susan was a very proper sort of person, and not one to discuss private matters. She glanced at Joyce, then smiled. "The Widgets?" She shook her head. "That phrase might be the most facetious term I've ever heard used to describe a serious situation, certainly in our family." She hesitated for a moment to gather her thoughts. "Robin has been having progressively worse monthly cycles. She suffers terribly from PMS, and in the last year it's gotten worse, much worse.

"The problem is affecting her work, and frankly I think her marriage could be in jeopardy if something isn't done. Nothing seems to work. She turns into another woman. It's worse than you might imagine, since you've only ever seen one side of her personality."

I could plainly see that Susan wasn't over-reacting, not this lady. These people had a serious problem.

I glanced at Joyce. "We're so sorry that she has to deal with such a serious case of PMS. How long has it been noticeable?"

Susan said, "It started, maybe four or five years ago, but it's so much more serious now. It's as if each month we all start to prepare for a siege, and we dread it."

"Well, what does her Doctor say? There are all sorts of products being touted for the 'Syndrome.'"

Susan laughed. "Her M.D. has been our family doctor for 35 years, and he's recommended everything you can imagine. His own daughter is going through the same thing. It's just terrible for some women!"

We ordered more coffee. "Susan, I know Joyce has told you how interested I am in this problem, and I assume that's why you decided to include me. I'm really glad you did. You know, it's strange but as common as PMS is, I've never seen anyone suffering all-out from it. I might have seen them, but I didn't know it."

Susan said, "I imagine most women try to hide it, especially from you, being here and all."

Joyce said, "That's true. Some talk to me about it, but they don't want others to know."

Susan said, "That's why you haven't seen Robin. I talked her into coming in the hope that you and Joyce might think of something, and talk to her. She loves the baths so much."

I got the picture. "Susan, the bottom line is this: I read in magazines about several products that supposedly treat the symptoms of PMS and I'm sure that those products work for a lot of women. Those companies can tell you how their products are *supposed* to work. Now whether they do, or not is another story.

"It's kind of like migraines. Every health magazine advertises all kinds of cures for migraines. I think sometimes that if the products really worked as well as they said they would, we wouldn't have any PMS or migraines."

I added, "You know, the clay does so much, and things are going so well, if we talk too much about some of these areas it makes us look like snake-oil salesmen."

"Snake oil my foot!" Susan said. She pointed to her arthritic feet. "And look at Larry, Jr's face. You can't imagine how many different remedies we tried before we found your clay for his face! That boy should be working here. He loves the clay."

I said, smiling, "He's a Disciple."

Susan said, "Oh, yes, that's what you call us!"

We all laughed. "Well, how do we start with Robin?"

I offered a suggestion. "Joyce has a lot of experience with this problem, and women talk to her. She has a way about her."

Joyce said, "Cano, you said the next time something happened like this, you wanted a written record."

"Yes, it could mean a lot some day. I mean there's so many women who suffer from the syndrome, it could be a real benefit."

Susan said, "I'm so glad we talked. How will we approach the subject?"

"There's your gal." I pointed to Joyce.

Joyce picked up right away. "It's just a matter of utilizing the clay four to five days before and then through her cycle. She'll be drinking clay water first thing in the morning and last thing at night. Since she doesn't sleep well, I'll have her nightly soak in a bath of warm to hot clay water, and at the same time apply a hot clay soaked washcloth to her face and the nape of her neck."

Susan was encouraged. "Oh, that sounds wonderful!"

Joyce added, "I'll be glad when we can prove that the ultimate benefit of clay therapy is to proactively stop the source of the problem, rather than dealing reactively with the effects. You can look forward to some degree of relief and possibly help short-circuit the whole problem."

I was proud of Joyce.

Joyce turned to me. "You know, more and more I sense we should recommend our clay to prevent problems before they start. That will ultimately be the great benefit."

I felt complimented that Susan had confided in us about

something so important to her family. I left a few hours later for Los Angeles. I had to keep the wheels oiled that caused the whole thing to function.

A few months later, on a Saturday morning, I had breakfast at the Denny's restaurant directly across from the Mirage Hotel.

As I stood in line to pay my check, someone tapped me on the shoulder and asked, "Aren't you Cano Graham, from the Crystal Cross?"

I loved it, and smiled at the introduction. "Yes, I am. What's up?"

He laughed from the inside out. "Mr. C., we love ya man! We all love ya! My wife Robin, my mom Susan, my son Larry, Jr. and me. I'm Larry, Sr.! You cleared our house of widgets! The widgets are a thing of the past. My mom's arthritis is much better, and just look at Larry, Jr.!"

There in a booth sat Susan, Robin, and Larry, Jr. waving and smiling. Robin looked beautiful! My lady had four more Disciples!

ෆ   ෆ   ෆ

We don't know how this clay works on PMS, but it does, and fast. The menstrual period puts in motion a lot of hormones and physiological reactions. Sometimes things get out of line. Some circuits short-circuit or electrical impulses misfire. The controls jam, and the nerves start screaming. The brain and body start over-reacting to some signals, and that sets in motion a reaction that gets out of sync with the body's natural internal order.

But, all the explanations together don't amount to a hill of beans to the women who suffer from PMS! I've gotten more hugs from new Clay Disciples because of this clay's ability to counter PMS than anything else, and that's a great pay off!

Chapter 19

Leroy

It is the heart always that sees, before the head can see.

Thomas Carlyle

Sometimes, we can never forget the first impression that a person makes on us. On the other hand, I know of cases where the opposite holds true, when the last impression is the one etched forever on our memory. With Leroy, it's both.

I had just finished doing another radio show in Las Vegas. Joyce, Ruthie, and Sylvia had put together an impromptu party. It all felt like a holiday for our locals and new clients as well. Locals brought food, wine flowed, and we were on a roll. I counted twenty people in the front room and kitchen. Then Leroy made his appearance. Seems the smell of all that food was more than he could take. I saw him first as he poked his head in the door.

Leroy, a big old black Labrador retriever, made quite an impression on those who saw him. Once you saw him, you knew that he had been a boss dog for a long time. But, time had taken its toll. His tail still curved proudly over his back, (the sign of a dominant dog), but arthritis in his back hips and legs caused him to almost pull himself by his front paws. When he stuck his head inside to check out the appetizing smells and other possibilities, he suddenly drew back because something outside had captured his attention. Sitting in my recliner, I had a clear view of what happened next.

He stood on the porch, watching several local dogs following along behind a city dog that was in season. She was giving the local country boys a real thrill, but I could see Leroy making the scene in his imagination through memories of the alpha male that he had once been. He glanced one more time wistfully at the scene before him, and turned to complete his entry into the kitchen.

I like dogs, but I loved Leroy, even though we hadn't been formally introduced. I was relaxed, and becoming more fascinated by Leroy with every wag of his tail. I sensed that Leroy had a plan. Old dogs remind me of old men. They're not smarter than the younger guys; they just know exactly what they can get away with in a given situation.

Leroy stood there letting folks pat him on the head and tell him what a good-boy he was. His nose was in the air, determining the location of everything of gustatory interest to him. He had no interest in the cake or potato salad. Beans didn't interest him. He was on the lookout for the hard stuff, the main line. He knew there were distractions with everyone talking, and telling their clay stories. He again raised his head like a bird dog on point, when he caught the aroma and sight of a large slab of corned beef about to be served.

I thought, oh no! No Leroy, don't do it! He put his head close to the table, and pulled his backside along like a person with crutches will pull a lame leg along. He slowly scanned the room from side to side to see if the coast was clear, in the furtive manner of a bold bank robber. I was witnessing a full-blown robbery, but in this case it was a deft corned beef heist in progress.

I thought, oh my God, he's going to do it! I thought for sure that someone would drag the booty away, out of his reach, before he could make good on his intentions. But Leroy knew from experience that wasted motion could screw up a good plan. He drew closer, determined to complete the act. He looked around.

Everyone stayed busy, blissfully unaware of his plan.

Now! He had one big paw on a chair, and in one black blur of motion, he was up and had the whole slab of meat in his mouth. No walking it outside for Leroy! No time! At that microsecond, he glanced at me watching him at work. He knew I knew.

Someone screamed, "That dog just ate the whole corned beef! All of it!"

A little old lady scolded him. "Bad dog!"

Leroy looked up at her as if to say, "So? It's all gone. No big deal. What are you going to do, put me in jail?"

She shook a finger close to his nose and repeated, "Bad dog!"

Leroy looked at me as if to say, "Give me break," then he calmly dropped his big head, and began to pull himself outside. I loved it!

"What's his name?"

"Leroy. He's a hell of a dog, but he's about through now. They're going to put him to sleep soon."

I asked, "How old is he?"

"Thirteen years. He's had a long run. You should hear the stories that people tell about his escapades."

"I just saw one that tells me a lot. That dog's got more guts than a Chicago slaughterhouse."

Someone said, "Yeah, he's something."

He wasn't out the door yet, and I yelled across the room, "Leroy!" He turned to see who had called him in such a commanding fashion, and our eyes connected across the room. I had a glass of wine, and he had a stomach full of corned beef. Our cups were both full. He knew it was me, and stopped in his tracks.

I said, "Leroy, come here." I waved him over to me. "Come on, pal. No problem. Let's get acquainted. Come on over."

He wanted to lie down. He was full, tired and he was sort of put off by the other dogs chasing his dream girl through the streets without his approval.

He slowly ambled over. He walked with his head down a little to show humility and respect, very important when you get older. It's more of an affirmation of values than a demonstration of surrender.

When he got close I said, "It *sure* is good to meet you. I've heard about you. Why don't we get to know each other?"

He sat close now. He looked at me with understanding in those big, sad eyes, wagged his tail ever so slightly, and laid that big head of his in my lap. I enjoyed it as one of those rare moments when two souls meet, and realize that they love each other. Everyone in the room stood watching.

I leaned over, put my head down close to his and said, "I know you've been down many a road. You can stay here for as long as you want, and nobody is going to put you down next week."

He heaved a restful sigh. Labs have a trait of resting their heads on things. Yep, we just straight up loved each other.

I whispered when I told him, "Leroy, I've got a plan regarding that bad back and leg. It's arthritis, isn't it? I just wanted to meet you today. So get some rest, and tomorrow afternoon I'll get you started on some clay treatments."

I swear he understood every word I had said to him. I asked someone to bring me a bowl of water with a handful of clay in it. In just a minute, he had slurped up the clay water. I suggested that we put a spoonful of powdered clay in his food and water daily.

He went out on the porch, and lay down, resting his head on his paws. His head came up in a hurry though, when the city girl pranced by with her entourage in tow. They were getting busy. He was full and tired. He lay his big head back down, licked his lips, and let out a big sigh. Memories would have to do for now.

The next day, Sunday, Leroy knew something was up. I started the day off by giving him a good, thorough bath with clay water. I toweled him dry and let him in the house. I could tell he already felt better. He moved easier, faster, with less pain.

After a couple of hours, I covered his back and legs with the clay, making sure to surround the areas of discomfort really well. I knew one potential problem. The clay can be too cool if one is in the wind, or a breeze. So, I made sure that he kept warm. Also, I knew that when the clay started to dry that the pulling effect, the tightening sensation, would drive him bonkers. It does that to people, and people at least know what's happening so they can mentally adjust.

Sure enough, what I was afraid of happened. The clay started to dry and pull, and Leroy began to go nuts. I grabbed him up, carried him to an outside shower, and we proceeded to shower together.

After a few minutes I let him out of the shower and a customer yelled out, "He's walking! Leroy's walking!!"

There he was, just walking along as if he'd never had a problem. Then everyone began to chant, "Le-Roy! Le-Roy! Le-Roy!"

What a wonderful moment! Glorious! Magnificent! Inspiring! We realized that we had witnessed a remarkable demonstration of what the legendary clay could do. I let Leroy off the leash, and he made the rounds taking the petting and choruses of good boy! Then he stopped. He stood absolutely still, with his head up and his tail curled high over his back.

Suddenly, he started running through the people on the patio, and straight down the road to where the city girl held court. Leroy was gone all day long. He lived to be almost fifteen years old.

ଓ   ଓ   ଓ

My editor was doubtful that one treatment on a dog's arthritic hip would achieve such remarkable results. Send us a before and after video when you prove it on your own animal.

ଓ   ଓ   ଓ

Dear Lord, Let me be as good as my dog thinks I am.

Chapter 20

The Escapees

To fill the hour, that is happiness; to fill the hour, and leave no crevice for a repentance or an approval.

Ralph Waldo Emerson

Curt popped his head through the office door. "Cano, I know you're about to leave for LA, but there's a man out here by the name of Daniels. Says he wants to see you."

I glanced out the window and saw a pickup truck full of Indians. I stepped outside and admired the scene of the central figure of the four generations sitting inside and outside that truck, a dignified gray-haired old Indian. He sat in the truck bed on a pile of heavy blankets, surrounded by a half dozen or so contented kids along with a couple of middle aged adults.

"Are you Cano Graham?"

I felt as though two-dozen sets of interested eyes were scrutinizing me.

I reached over the top of all those keen brown eyes and mops of shiny coal black hair, gently grasped his fingertips, and said, "Yes sir, Mr. Daniels, I am."

I scanned every confident young face, all offshoots of the handsome old man, and then met his eyes. I sensed that he thought well of anyone who naturally appreciated the children of his children's children. He struck me as a happy man. "Glad you're all here, how can I help you?"

The collection of quick brown eyes shifted to their great grandfather for his response.

"We have some common friends, one plays a mean fiddle and the other can make a tambourine dance."

The ice that never existed instantly broke.

I was rustling the hair of one restless ten-year-old boy when I got it. "Art and Luella Babbit are friends of yours? All right! Since that's the case, then I've just acquired a dozen new friends. Welcome to my place, Mr. Daniels."

The old patriarch said, "Art tells me you're interest in *EE-WAH-KEE.*"

"Art said what? EE what?

The beautiful old guy was having fun with me, and knowing I didn't yet understand, he quietly, politely, and still smiling said again, "*EE-WAH-KEE.*"

He knew by my expression that he had me. "Cano, Hmm, that's a strange name for a white man."

"Part white."

He grinned, "Yes, Art told me. Choctaw, from Oklahoma."

"Yes, with a few other things thrown in."

He gestured to include all the others and said, "We're Shoshone." He laughed. "Nothing else added. We live outside of Bishop. It's a long drive."

I still didn't know where this was all going for sure. "Sure is, a long, hot drive, but you're all here. Good, now about the *EE-WAH-KEE?*"

He helped me by phonetically sounding out the word, then said, "*EE-WAH-KEE.* That's what you got here. It's why we come. It means Earth Medicine, *EE-WAH-KEE.* This gray- green clay here is what many tribes call *EE-WAH-KEE.*"

"You don't say, well I'll be darned. I never heard that before. Art never mentioned it."

Mr. Daniels said, "I don't think Art knew it by that name. He came from far north."

"That makes sense. Anyway he knows about my interest. I see, now I understand. *EE-WAH-KEE.* Interesting. Well, you all get out and stretch your legs." I pointed to the pool area and said, "The restrooms are over there. Can you stay long?"

He simply said, "We come for the clay, for the day."

I like the way that sounded. I remembered thinking I had to make a note of that; Clay for the Day.

So, just that fast my plans changed. I'd planned on doing some business that afternoon in LA but I instantly altered those plans. I had to have my priorities.

"All right, good enough! Now, let's see …"

His daughter, sitting next to her husband in the cab helped me out by saying, "Mr. Graham, Art told us what we'd need. We've all got our swimsuits and we brought enough food and drinks for everyone including your workers, so we're all fixed up. If you'll just show us where to go?"

Joyce could see I needed help. She sauntered over, and I introduced her to everyone.

"Hi babe, this is Mr. Daniels' family. They're going to be here all day. They came for the Clay Pools. You know who their friends are? Art and Luella!"

The news delighted her. "Oh that's good to hear."

"Sure is! They've got everything they need: suits and food and lots of time."

Joyce said, "Why don't we get them a room so they can store the food and use the stove when they need it. She turned her attention to the two mothers and added, "There are two beds in the room so the little ones can nap if they get tired."

Three or four of the kids said, "We aren't gonna get tired."

Mr. Daniels watched the kids scramble out of the truck. "Art says you have day rates?"

"Mr. Daniels, you keep looking around. Have you been here

169

before?"

He grinned and said, "A long time ago. None of this was here back then."

"Oh? Well anyway, first off, please, don't even think about any type of rates for today. We don't have anything scheduled today. It'll be slow around here. We're actually closed this week so we can do some heavy landscaping. It's a good time to be here. We just finished our second clay pool. The place is a mess, but, frankly, you being Art's friends and all, well, today it would be my treat just to have your family here. I'm curious, you've used this clay before haven't you?"

He nodded. "Yes, and it's time for these old bones to enjoy it again."

"That's great. I'm more than compensated by sharing my place and the *EE-WHA-KEE* with you all. Have the kids ever been in clay before?"

"No, never. No one in the family but me."

"How long ago was that?"

He took off his old straw cowboy hat, pulled a worn blue bandana from his back pocket, wiped his brow, and pensively absorbed the sky and distant hills. "Long time ago. I was a boy with my father. My dad and his brother used to bring their families here after winter was over. We used to camp on the backside of that hill."

He pointed with his hat to the hill where the cross stood. "There's always been a white cross on that hill. Not that big though. The miners put it there to show where there was water." He put his hat back on, laughed, and said, "Indians didn't need a cross."

He scratched his neck. "But the last time I remember using or playing in the clay was because of my grandfather, he had sore knees and ankles. The old fellow could hardly walk. He was the main reason we all came. Back then there was nothing here, no building, just some tents set up by a few miners."

170

I loved his story. "How old were you?"

He pointed at an eight- or nine-year-old-boy and said, "About his age."

"You were a little boy, and you remember?"

"Sure do." He pointed toward the hill and the Cross and said, "I remember us kids climbing that hill, and seeing who could throw rocks the farthest. The land hasn't changed much at all. I was in Tecopa twenty or so years ago, in the late 60s or maybe it was the early 70s, for a few days. It seemed a lot busier then. I guess when the miners pulled out everyone moved away. But you know, I never again heard of anyone using the clay. I used to wonder about it. When Art told me what you were doing, I knew I wanted to come down."

"Did you always live up by Bishop?"

"Oh, no. All my family came from up north of Las Vegas, up by Utah. I've just lived in Bishop for seven years. I moved there to live with my daughter after their mother died."

I motioned to all his family and said, "Looks like you have enough to keep you busy. You're a lucky man."

The drive down had taken its toll on him. He looked tired when he said, "Yes, yes, I know, and thank you, Mr. Graham."

I certainly liked this man and felt complimented that what I created had attracted him. "Mr. Daniels, you said you could spend the day? Where do you intend to spend the night?"

"We're driving back home tonight."

"Mr. Daniels, let me suggest something. Stay here, on the house. We're slow. We have no reservations, no guests. If the sawing and hammering don't bother you, well, we'd be glad to have you all."

He fumbled with his straw hat and said, "Thanks Mr. Graham, but I'd planned to leave here about 6:00 or so this evening."

"I wish you'd reconsider. I mean that would put you in Bishop about 10:30. We've got plenty of room, and the kids will get a big kick out of spending the night. You can leave early tomorrow morning while it's still cool. As you well know, crossing Death Valley tonight will still be plenty miserable. That's too far after a full day here."

"Mr. Graham, that's mighty nice of you to go to the trouble of putting up with all these kids and all of us."

"Now, Mr. Daniels, it will be my pleasure. I need a change of pace, and these kids will definitely change our pace. In fact, I can't wait to call Art and Luella and several others so we can have a little get together tonight, right here!"

"Art told me it might be like this. If you were in town."

"Sure enough. It'll be fun! I enjoy kids. They're a break for me." A plan was already taking shape. "I can make up some ghost stories that'll keep 'em up half the night."

He laughed at the prospect.

Then he said with a sly wink, "One more thing: Art, Luella, and me used to put on a pretty good show with them doing what they do and me playing my harmonica."

"You play a harmonica?"

"All night if need be, and I never leave home without it."

We were already having a good time, and some of the kids were hanging around, getting a kick out of watching their great grandfather laughing and enjoying himself. Those kids had a night coming they wouldn't soon forget, nor would any of us adults.

Next I called Art. "Hey Big Guy! There's a friend of yours and some of his family here at my place. They're going to spend the day and night."

"Friends of mine?"

"Yep, good friends too, I'd imagine.

"Says he can keep up with you and Luella all night."

Art laughed and said, "A doin' what?"

"Says he'll be playing a smooth harmonica."

"A harmonica? Yeeeow! Bob Daniels is there? Lordy, Lord bar the doors! Cano, you gonna be in town tonight?"

"Arthur, I wouldn't miss this one for the world!"

"You say some of his family, who? Is his daughter there?"

"I don't know the names, but they're a beautiful bunch. Classy! I've never seen so many dark brown eyes in such close quarters."

Art moaned. "I once saw hers in close quarters. Oh my, this could be a good one."

"Art, can you pull everyone together who would enjoy a spur of the moment party for Mr. Daniels?"

"Cano, Bob's got several friends here among the older set. He hasn't been down this way in years. Let's see, Beulah, Sylvia, lemme see, Ruthie, Mori. I know some folks in Death Valley and I know of some in Pahrump would love to see him. You know he was a pure champion bronco rider in his day. You could have a full house."

"That's great, we'll do it in the recreation room Curt just finished. That'll be plenty big enough."

"How many has he got with him?"

"Must be seven or so under twelve years old and four adults. How many will you get here?"

"Oh, a dozen or so for sure. Bob has lots of friends, and a pretty daughter. She once came to see me fight in Reno. You say he has two daughters there? Hmmm, only has two! One of 'em must be her."

"Art, what weight did you fight at?"

"One forty-seven."

"You were small."

"Light and fast. And so was she!"

"Well, Art, things change. She's not petite now, real sweet, also pleasingly plump."

"Luella will no doubt notice and appreciate that fact."

"I hope you survive the night."

"Me too." He bellowed a huge belly laugh.

"Art why don't we ask them all to be here around 8:00 or so. That'll give everyone a chance to have their dinner, and for things

173

to cool off a bit. I told Mr. Daniels that this afternoon we'd turn the kids all loose in the clay pools. He's really looking forward to that scene. After the clay I'll turn the swimming pool over to 'em all. It should be a full day."

"I didn't realize Bob knew so much about the clay until we talked. He used it when he was a boy with his father."

"Yes, he told me. It was a long time ago."

"By the way Art, Joyce and I plan to take the kids up on the hill around sundown. I'm gonna have the workers bring wood up for a fire. We'll roast some marshmallows, and I'll tell 'em some ghost stories that'll curl that long black hair up tight."

"Are you gonna give 'em the Crystal Bowl Treatment?"

"You're reading my mind again. Sure enough! I'll have someone make the thing whine real good."

"Cano, you'll scare the hell outta those kids."

"That's the idea. Michael can make some of the spookiest sounds I ever heard with that bowl. He knows just how to rub it with that rubber thing. Anyway, the weird sounds of that big crystal bowl will carry those kids to another zone. I've got an idea. I'm gonna tell 'em about a headless hermit that comes out of the hills on some nights and just wanders around looking for a head to fit on his shoulders."

"Cano! Where do you come up with this stuff? It sounds better than us a playing music."

With Art's encouragement I got into the idea a little more. "Yeah, it'll be fun. Okay, let's see. I'm going to tell them that he can't talk because he hasn't got a head. Are you there, Art?"

"Yea, I'm here. But where are the kids going to be after you start this." He started to laugh.

"How about this Art? Okay, he hasn't got a head, and all he does is moan and wail because he's hungry all the time."

Art jumped in. "I know, cause he's got no head, he can't eat, and they'll be afraid he'll catch them and eat 'em all up?"

"Right! Then about that time I'll signal for our help to really make that bowl howl like crazy."

"Hell fire man, you're making the hair stand up on my neck, and it's the middle of the day and I'm on the phone."

"Great! So you think it'll work?"

"Work? My God man! They'll be palefaces by the time they come down off the hill."

We all have those unforgettable nights that we file away with our memories, and this was to be one of those special times. The older folks loved seeing Bob Daniels with his family and talking about what used to be, and listening to the music that reminded them of when they would play all night long.

I added a bit more spice to the evening for the young ones by having one of Curt's crew cover himself with a flowing sheet and appear like a floating vision just beyond the fire's light. This created the effect of the headless one floating about the sand and rock preparing to pounce on the first little Indian he could catch off guard. They all seemed to bunch up close to me and stayed very much on guard. Their fear magnified when the player of the big crystal bowl heightened the ambient symphony of eerie, haunting, spooky sounds that seemed to come from the bowels of the earth and the stars at the same time.

By the time we decided to make a break for safety, and escape from the headless hermit's clutches, we were almost goners. Those kids actually kicked up a dust cloud racing frantically down the hill. The waiting hot chocolate and cookies soothed some jangled nerves. The Escapees were convincing as they related to their parents and great grandfather the perils of the wonderful night.

ᴄ8 ᴄ8 ᴄ8

Children have never been very good at listening to their elders, but they have never failed to imitate them.

James Baldwin

Chapter 21

The Mothers Are Gone

The essence of pleasure is spontaneity.　　　　Germaine Greer

Robert came from a very wealthy family, working in one of the hottest little towns in the United States, in the most miserable conditions, exposed daily to noxious fumes that kicked up his allergies. Yet, he did this with a poise and attitude that inspired everyone around him, a real delight. Husky, with black hair and eyes to match, he had one of those natural smiles that framed beautiful teeth. He was also a one-man public relations firm for the Crystal Cross Therapeutic Clay Center. He loved to say, "I got you a bunch last week. Did they tell you I sent 'em up?"

Now Baker, California is only fifty miles from Tecopa Hot Springs, yet many tourists had no idea we existed or what we did, but they did know after Robert got through with his spiel about the place.

I ran through all these thoughts about Robert as I roared off of I-15 and sort of coasted into Baker. I had a lot of friends in Baker, but Robert was my favorite. He was on duty and waving me into position for gas as if I were a racecar heading for the pit.

"Hi Cano, the works?" He always asked that, I think that was his way of saying, "I got everything covered, go get some coffee."

"Hi Bud, you're looking good. How's the lady treating you?"

He grinned wide when he said, "She loves me, she just straight up loves me. She keeps me outta trouble and clean."

The first time I saw Robert he was struggling and I was preoccupied with some unimportant and mundane thoughts of my own.

One very hot day, I was in a hurry and edgy about something, terribly important, I'm sure, when I noticed he didn't look well. He was leaning on a pole next to a pump with his head cradled by his fingers.

He didn't even look up when he said to me, "Okay, that'll be $20.50."

He looked so tired, and from the way he squinted his eyes, I could tell he was having a bad day.

I gave him the $20.50 and said, "Thanks," and got into my truck.

He asked, "Aren't you the man from Tecopa that has the Clay place?"

I nodded and hit the starter. I was ready to roll.

He wiped his face with a wet towel. Something seemed very wrong. I placed the gear in drive but didn't start to move. My foot was on the brake. I glanced at him again, something was just wrong with this picture.

I shifted into park so I could give him my undivided attention. "What's wrong with you?"

He squeezed a wet towel over his head and took a deep breath, let it out, then wiped his face again. "Headache, bad damn headache."

"Do you get 'em often?"

He nodded. "More all the time, and these sores, they hurt. They drive me nuts when I sweat and they sting. I'm messed up big time!"

He pulled the neck of his T-shirt down to show me four or five sores on his neck and shoulders. They looked oozy and miserable.

I remembered that I had seen a man at my place that had

worked in a plant of some kind in Las Vegas who had these same symptoms. He called it a chemical injury from exposure to toxic fumes. The clay had worked on him so well that his foreman had come to see for himself what it was all about. At about that same time I began to realize how common this sort of thing might be.

"Do you have many of those sores on the rest of your body?"

He turned around and pulled his T-shirt up over his shoulders so I could see his bare back. If they felt as bad as they looked, well, this young man had a serious problem.

"Do you know what causes them?" I asked.

He said, "It's this damn place. It's hot." He pointed above his head. "The cover over all the gas pumps sort of keeps the fumes trapped. I got to find different work. It's not every day, but when it's like this with no wind blowing, man it's too much."

At that time, I had only ever seen three people with those specific problems. Now we call it Multiple Chemical Sensitivity, though I didn't know of that definition at the time.

"Come up to my place and spend some time when you can take off for a day, a full day."

"Tomorrow. It's not my day off, but I can make arrangements to come up. I'll bring my wife and baby." Then he stuck his hand in the window to me and said, "My name is Robert."

"Hi, I'm Cano Graham."

He asked, "Are you Mexican? That's a Mexican name."

"No," I said, "It's a name that was hung on me twenty years ago by some Mexican-Indian kids. It just stuck."

"Means gray," he said, "It's because of your hair."

I said, "Right."

"What time tomorrow?" "Oh, about ten o'clock, how's that for you?"

"Fine. We'll enjoy the day. You're going to use that clay stuff on me, aren't you?"

"Yep, I sure am. I have reason to believe it'll do you a lot of good."

"See ya tomorrow, Robert."

ଔ   ଔ   ଔ

He always wore a plantation style hat and sunglasses so that when he arrived with his wife and new baby he had the appearance of a tourist a thousand miles from home. I gave him an outline of what to do that day and instructed the manager to see to it that he got the whole treatment and that when he left he had ample clay to treat himself at home. Eight days later, I pulled into Baker once again and wondered about Robert. He saw me before I even pulled into the station. He was wearing a good-looking big new hat, neat sunglasses, and a new white T-shirt and crisp jeans. Before I got within a hundred feet of the pumps he whipped off the big hat then the T-shirt and sunglasses. He had the build of a football player and he grinned that big grin and held his arms over his head with his head back and yelled, "Yes! Yes! Yes!"

I pulled up closer. "I take it things are better?"

He started showing off a bit, twisting to a melody only he could hear and shouted, "Better? Those mothers are gone, gone, gone! *No más, nada, vamoos.* Free at last, free at last!"

I got out of the truck, and Robert gave me a big hug.

Many years have passed since I last saw Robert. Some day, he and many others may read this account of my experiences at the Crystal Cross Therapeutic Clay Center. If it says anything about those times it's simply that I love you all. We shared something so very special.

Chapter 22

The Dirty Deed

Comedy is the last refuge of the nonconformist mind.
Gilbert Seldes

Tired and sleepy, I really shouldn't have been driving, but I had to get back to Tecopa Hot Springs. The usual soft rock on the radio wasn't working. I needed something else, something different, to keep me awake. Then I saw them, three guys on the road ahead of me hitchhiking. Between two youngsters, who looked like runaways, a small, thin, older man stoically waited for a ride. I chose the little older fellow.

He looked harmless enough with a neat traveling bag at his feet, a book clutched in his left hand, and his right thumb held high in the air. He topped this off with a huge sun hat that seemed to ride on his ears. Ah! This wasn't the first time on the road for him. Even from a distance he had the bearing of a seasoned traveler.

I pulled up next to my chosen one, leaned over towards him, and was about to ask how far he was going when he poked his head through the open window, thrust a big Bible at me, and with eyes flashing yelled, "Praise the Lord!"

Well Hell! The last thing I wanted was a Bible-thumping companion to chitchat with, but on the other hand, the casting just might be perfect. I decided to play it out. Improvisation is the key to discovering those wonderful spontaneous moments that can never be written. Instinctively I drew back when his arm and shoulder appeared inside the cab.

I thought, "Christ! I've got a live one!"

Before I could gather my wits and consider the options, my fiery little new acquaintance blurted out: "Sir! Do you know Christ died for your sins?"

The degree of certainty in his voice had me blinking in defense when without forethought my sinful lips gasped, "Oh, no! I'm so sorry, I didn't know he was sick!"

He jerked back, stunned as if he had been hit with some kind of electric theological overload.

At that point I caught the unmistakable odor of what I suspected. My little traveling evangelist was drunk as a skunk, and flying high with the angels of the Good Book on his side! He gathered up his bag, himself, and started to open the door saying, "No sir, he wasn't sick, I mean..."

I stopped the little guy by holding up my hand like a traffic cop and said in my friendliest manner, "Sir, excuse me, but it's rather crowded in here right now." I pointed to the empty passenger seat. "As you can see. I'm teaching my friend here how to drive this truck, and the fact is, well, I must apologize. We're having an awfully heated discussion concerning gay rights. I mean, he doesn't like my position on that subject, plus he really hates me for smoking grass. I wonder just how do you feel about those issues?"

He considered his answer. "Well, Mister, I don't know for sure."

I helped him out by changing the conversation back to the original issue. "Oh! That's okay never mind. Anyway I think you'd find it far too crowded for three of us in here, but that's not to say you're not welcome to sit between us. I pointed to the back. "Or possibly ride in the truck bed if you'd like. I mean, it's up to you."

He poked his head inside the cab again, and with anxious childlike eyes said, "Sir, there's someone else here now? Right now?"

I smiled as if I didn't understand his question. "Why certainly he's here! Oh Yes! You're only a few inches from his ear in fact."

He jerked back to see what wasn't there.

I continued, "He's here all right. I slipped into a more personal tone and confided, "He's such a terrible driver. Can't seem to get the hang of it. You know what I mean?"

Bless his heart. He stepped back and scanned the fast moving freeway as if searching for an alternate route, or even counsel to assist with this decision. Then under his whispered breath escaped the words, "Help me Lord!" Then louder he asked, "I don't know, are you driving or is a-ah-he?"

At this point I couldn't tell if he was stalling or praying. I reassured him by saying, "Oh, I am, at least most of the time."

"Most of the time?"

I nodded. "Well, nice talking to you, but we must be going, so what would you like to do?"

He searched the highway again for direction. "Ah, yes, sir I don't want to bother you and your friend. I'll be fine back here." He gently placed his bag in the truck bed, and carefully crawled over the tailgate.

I opened the back window. "Okay, are you ready?"

He nodded. "Also, a word of warning. Don't mind my friend's foul language. We argue a lot, and he cusses like a drunken sailor."

He nodded his head fast in short jerks making his hat quiver.

I sensed he wasn't too secure with the hasty decision to ride with me on this trip, but that concern was soon history because ready or not, we were quickly up to cruising speed.

One must play these improvised scenes moment to moment, because anything too structured doesn't work well and becomes flat. I decided to simply go with my normal flow. I did what I had done a hundred times before. I locked my cruise control at 65, turned up the radio, sat sideways a bit, put my right arm over the seat, the left one out the window to play with the wind, and settled back guiding the truck with my left knee under the steering wheel.

I glanced in the rear view mirror, and saw what I expected. My passenger, sitting up and very alert, could plainly see the steering wheel move, but no hands on the wheel. I held up a gallon jug of water and asked if he cared for a cool drink. He refused. He had his own, and dove headfirst into the travel bag and extracted a half-pint of something to do the job he needed done. After he had a big pull of his medicine, he held it up offering me a taste.

I yelled back, "No thanks, the stuff makes me weird."

The little fella's expression seemed to say that he didn't need further proof.

I let things settle for a mile or so before I tried to take the wheel from my invisible passenger. The ungrateful student slapped my hand. Well, I slapped him back! I started screaming and cussing the hard-to-see lout and returned his action blow for blow, all the while cruising along with my knee doing the steering.

The little guy took another swig and crouched lower in the bed holding onto the side of the truck bed with one hand and the tailgate with the other. The scene was going well when I swerved a bit for special effect, and traded several more wild blows with my phantom friend.

My arms flew in all directions when I increased the tempo by becoming frantic and yelling, "You damn fool! Take your hands off the steering wheel! You'll get us all killed!"

By now, we had come up on a big semi rig loaded with something heavy and covered with a tarp. I knew my antics had alarmed my little passenger, but didn't think he'd do anything silly. Still, he might in his condition. I swerved back and forth from slow lane to fast lane, all the while flailing my arms and yelling, "Let Go! You'll kill us all!!" I eased into the fast lane and began to pass the semi. Surprise! The driver of the big rig must have thought I was very drunk or completely nuts, because he started leaning on his air horns and proceeded to scare the Hell out of me, and the Devil out of the little guy.

A few miles outside of Baker, I decided my new buddy had endured enough entertainment for the time being, so in the heat of yet another vicious struggle with you know who, I reached over, opened the passenger door and for all appearances kicked the invisible rascal out, and took visible control of my truck. I looked out the rear window as if to watch my invisible friend roll down the highway.

At that point, my guest in back turned to see if he could locate the tumbling body. I then made eye contact with my now quite sober little friend, and made the universal gesture for cutting someone's throat. I snarled fiendishly, and waved a last goodbye to the invisible one.

The dirty deed was done.

Within a minute or so I coasted into Baker, and as usual, found Robert on duty at the 76 station. He waved me in like my own private pit crew. "Hey Cano, the works?"

"Hi, Robert, yeah please, check it out. Whew! I've been busy. You'll need to get a rag. There's some blood on the front seat. I just had one hell of a fight. Almost got us killed!"

"What the…?" Robert was dumbfounded, "With who?"

My very sober passenger standing in the truck bed offered, "Oh he's right son, Lord knows it was a terrible thing to see, fighting for the wheel and all, almost got us all killed! I didn't think we'd make it. I was praying hard!" He raised his arms and said thankfully, "Praise the Lord!"

I glanced at Robert and my expression told him not to respond. Then to the little fella I said, "You're sure right. About got killed. By the way, would you care for some coffee or something before we continue to Las Vegas?"

Robert couldn't take anymore. "Cano, you're going to Las Vegas, not to Tecopa?" I motioned for him to chill out.

In a most appreciative tone the little fella said, "Oh, maybe a cold soda or something like that, but-ah-no, I won't be going to Vegas just now."

"Well you're more than welcome to ride along."

"Mister?" He squinted and asked Robert, "Can you see him? I mean will I be able to really see him too? You know, like I see you, I mean..."

Robert, working quietly, began to catch on.

I responded to the little guy, "Well, no, he's kind of hard to see, but he's there for sure!"

My passenger jumped out of the truck bed and held his big hat, bag, and Bible when he said, "Oh Lord, I know he's there! No question, but are you teaching him to drive, like the other one?"

These were moot questions because he wasn't about to get in my truck again, not when he thought I was completely delusional, or worse, working with the Devil! Robert had to turn away so as not to blow the scene.

I continued, "As a matter of fact I am teaching him, the problem is, this fool likes to go 90 mph, and he doesn't see very well, but you're welcome."

He cut me off. "No, thanks, but, uh, I believe I'll stay here in Baker for awhile, might even spend the night." He sighed deeply, even gratefully. He looked around the small desert town and said, "Nice, pretty little place. Yes sir. Believe I'll just relax here for a spell. I've got some praying to do, some real thanks to give."

I asked, "What's your name?"

"Little Roy...Roy Jourdan."

"Fine, Roy, my name is Cano. Glad we met, real glad about meeting you."

"Thanks, Cano! I feel the same way." He flexed his shoulders and relaxed.

"You know, Little Roy, prayer is a mighty powerful thing, and you proved it."

He was so pleased. "Yep, sure did! We made it, even when it looked like you was losing."

"That's a fact, I'll never forget it. Never." I wasn't kidding.

"Oh, me neither." Then he looked up at the cloudless sky and said, "Thank ya, Jesus!"

I said, "Amen" and meant it.

Robert seemed to enjoy this encounter, but now in a different way.

"Hey, Robert, check everything out. Mr. Jourdan and I are gonna go have a nice lunch and maybe a cold beer."

"We are? Lunch and a beer?" He smiled for the first time since we started our trip.

I put my arm around his shoulder as we started walking toward the restaurant. "You know, Roy, I kinda think the Good Lord wants us to have lunch, a cold beer and get a little better acquainted."

The idea of a cold beer caused both of us to quicken our walking pace and for the little guy to offer his feelings rather like a genuine testament.

"You know, Mr. Cano, I think he does too, yes sir, I sure do."

愉 愉 愉

Mr. Jourdan and I had lunch, talked things over and had a few good laughs. The little fella didn't go to Las Vegas that evening. In fact three weeks would pass before he made it to that dream. He came to the Crystal Cross with me that afternoon, did some work for Joyce, and some painting for Curt before he hit the road again. The Lord has a unique messenger in Little Roy. Look around, I know he's spreading the word somewhere and he's probably traveling. Buy him a lunch and a beer and since he's hitchhiking, ask him about the strangest ride he ever had. You can believe it because the little guy isn't stretching the story.

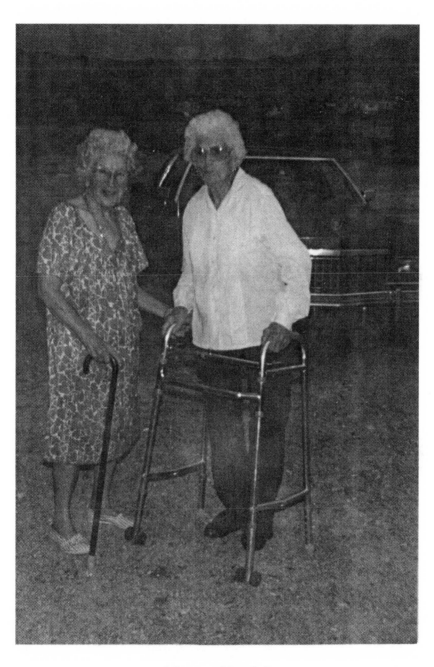

Mom and Buelah

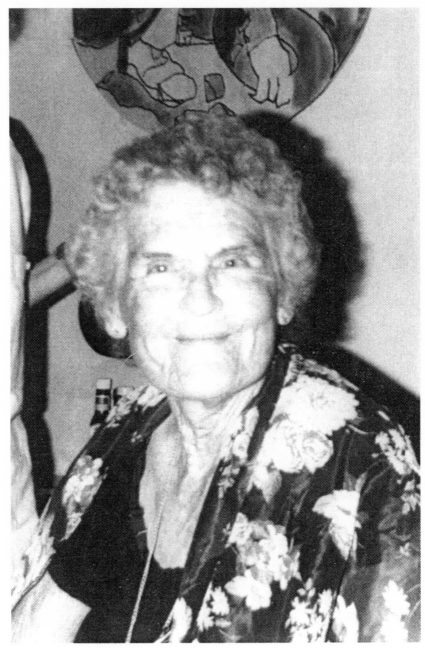

Sylvia

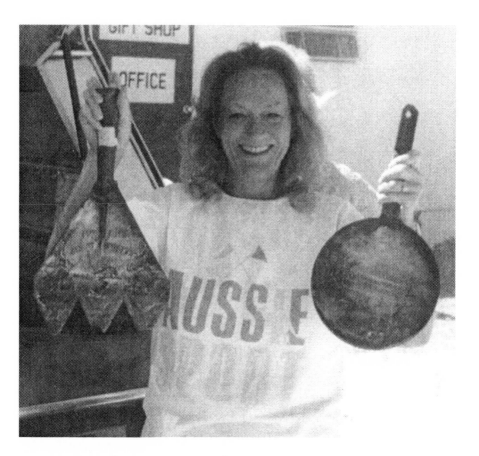

Joyce

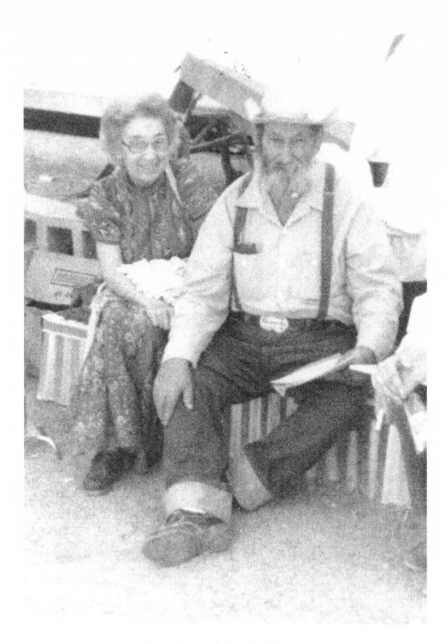

Louella and Art Babbit

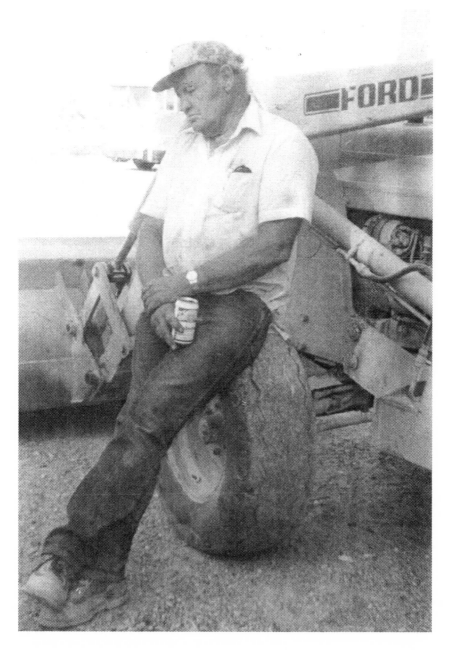

Curt

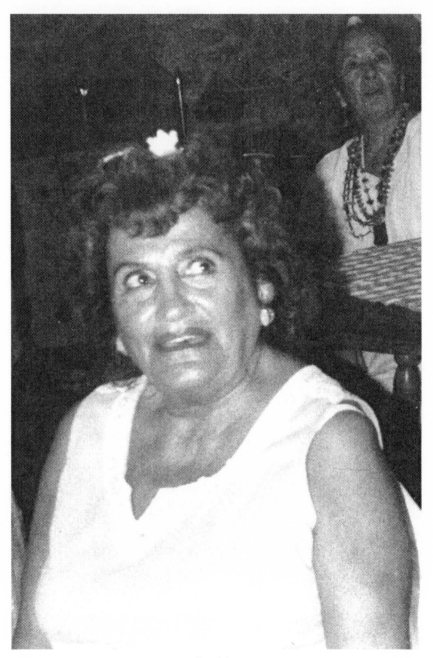

Ruthie

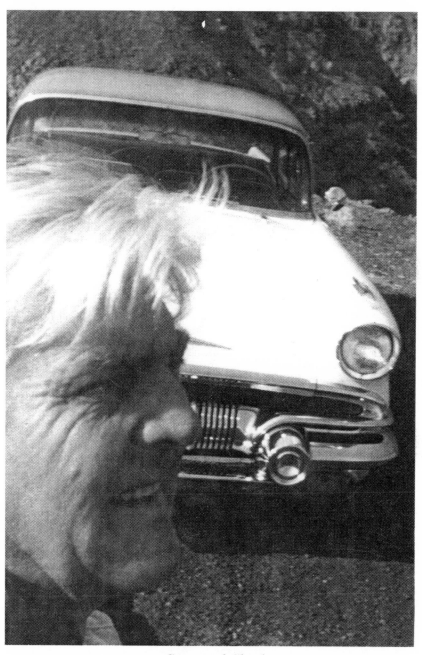

Cano and Chief

Chapter 23

Cindy

There's nothing so real in life as the things you've done…
inexorably, unalterably done. Sara Teasdale

The broken down, rattling vehicle spewed choking dust, tore into the parking lot, and caused rocks to fly like shrapnel. Skidding to a stop, Michael jumped out and slammed the door shut. It sounded like a crowbar smashing into a tub full of bottles. One thing for sure, he was in too much of a hurry.

Michael and his girlfriend Cindy took care of the place sometimes when we were gone, and he enjoyed certain liberties.

This evening he burst into the front room and yelled, "Cano, I need to use your truck!"

It wasn't like Michael to ask for the use of my truck.

"I'm thinking she may be in serious trouble."

I waved him down and pleaded, "Slow down, Mike. What are you talking about? Who's in trouble? Will you settle down?"

Mike was bright enough, but scared, big time.

Hearing all the racket, Joyce threw on a robe then joined us in the front room. I asked Michael to please start at the beginning.

He drew an impatient breath, brushed back his long hair, and tried hard to be cool. He lit a cigarette, and took a deep drag. "Okay, here it is. You know Cindy has been sick?"

I glanced at Joyce and said, "Yes, we thought it was the flu or something."

He shouted, "No Cano, she's got Toxic Shock Syndrome!"

"Say what? Toxic Shock? What's he talking about?" I turned to Mike, "Slow down and talk to me like you're sane, or you're outta' here!"

Mike buried his face in his hands. "Okay, I'm sorry. A few days ago she was real sick, and I took her to Valley Hospital in Las Vegas. She was diagnosed with Toxic Shock Syndrome. Cano, she was real sick.

"They put her on antibiotics, and then yesterday she started to get worse. I took her to the Death Valley Clinic because it's close, and my truck wasn't running too good. Anyway, the doctor there confirmed that she had Toxic Shock Syndrome. He checked her out real good, and scared the hell out of both of us! What an ass! After he examined her, he told us that she had lesions, and all the other symptoms of Toxic Shock, and that she'd be lucky to be alive in twenty-four hours! He really told her that. I heard him! Can you imagine?"

"Mike, take it easy! What happened next?"

"He wanted to see her again tomorrow morning, but she's getting worse tonight and they ain't open. She's sweating hard and has chills. Her color is bad, and she's throwing up the antibiotics as fast as they hit her stomach. I need to take her to Las Vegas now! She's bad! She can't wait 'til tomorrow! The pills ain't working, and she's getting worse. That's why I need your truck."

Joyce and I realized we needed to see for ourselves just what was going on. We dressed quickly. Joyce found my glasses, and we followed Mike out the door to his place.

"Just what the hell is Toxic Shock Syndrome and how bad is it?"

Joyce said, "I haven't heard much about it for the past few years, but it's a dangerous infection that some women get from using tampons. I don't remember much more than that. Anyway, I haven't heard about it lately."

"Didn't I read some time back that it could be fatal?"

She nodded. "Oh yes, it's bad. Very dangerous."

In a few minutes we arrived onto a very spooky set. The room was almost dark. Only one small table lamp was on, and it cast weird shadows around the room. I saw a mattress on the floor. As my eyes adjusted to the dim light, I found Cindy sitting on an old, overstuffed chair. She looked like an entirely different person.

Bloated, and sweating profusely, she had the look of someone fighting a severe bout of nausea. But the look of her eyes upset me the most. They seemed to bulge from her head in utter terror.

I felt like an animal trapped in a corner. I knew a lot about Clay Therapy, but never found myself in such a dangerous situation, with only the clay to depend on. In this case, we could see her getting worse by the minute.

Mike was out of his head.

I pulled Joyce aside. "Okay, what do I do? If I see this situation correctly, the decision has already been made for us. I mean, first off, do you feel that she's as sick as she appears?"

"Cano, I'm frightened. I know Cindy, she's in bad shape, and getting worse fast. If she's in Toxic Shock, I mean I've read how deadly it is, and that stupid doctor told her that she'd be lucky to be alive in twenty-four hours? Well, he's a cold ass alright, but I also remember an article saying that Toxic Shock Syndrome kills rapidly."

"I had planned on getting gas in Shoshone tomorrow. I know my truck probably doesn't have more than two gallons left. I bet I wouldn't get all the way to Pahrump. That alone stops me. We've got to do something, and quick!

"What if we made a run for it and ran out of gas at this time of night? The other thing, those antibiotics, she's throwing them up. Nothing about this makes it worth gambling her life on trying something that by all odds won't work. We've got to get fluids in her and at least try to counter the problem."

"We've got to try the clay. I mean it's our only shot. For sure it won't hurt her, and it might even neutralize the poisoning and stabilize her long enough to get to the doctor tomorrow.

"Okay, Babe let's roll. We've got to get our clay in her, and on her. Let's do it."

I had a small bucketful of gelled clay, and a sack of the dry powder in the truck. I was excited, like being in combat. I told Mike to get the clay from the truck, and bless his heart, he stopped to ask if we should try to get more antibiotics down her.

"No, no more. Get a pitcher of water and put a half-dozen tablespoons of our clay in it. Stir it with a wooden spoon."

Mike looked at me. "I know not to put a metal spoon in it. Damn!"

Mike knew about clay. He knew a lot about it, but this was his Cindy and he was worried sick.

I got Cindy to drink the first cup of clay water without a problem. Great! She didn't throw up. I then covered her upper body with the gelled clay, thankful that I had it with me and ready to use!

She began to cool down quickly. She drank more clay water and began to perceptibly relax. All this happened in a short period of time, something like fifteen to twenty minutes. Cindy was still in serious trouble, but she definitely looked better, not worse.

I visualized the clay absorbing all the antibiotics and poisons from her system. The topical application worked from the outside in, cooling her down, and also drawing out toxins. But the core toxic problem remained and that thought made me catch my breath.

I suggested that Mike make four large poultices to cover her abdominal area, and he was to then place them on her every two hours or so during the night. But something was missing. We needed to directly attack the area where the poison was coming from.

I didn't think that just flushing the area with a clay solution would be strong enough. I directed Michael to apply a series of poultices on her abdomen, while I thought about how to get the powdered clay directly to the source of the problem to soak up all the toxins.

I asked Mike to find a nylon stocking, and put a wooden spoon in it. I then poured approximately half a cup of the dry, powdered clay into the stocking. I asked Mike and Cindy to use the spoon handle to work the stocking deep into her vagina, and then remove the spoon. I asked that the clay stocking rig stay inserted until the following morning. When it was done, and Cindy was resting, Joyce and I left.

The next day, Mike and Cindy reported that the first poultice had a putrid odor to it, the second wasn't as bad, and the last ones were even better. She had started responding in a positive manner from the very start just by drinking the clay water, and the restorative effects didn't stop throughout the night. Cindy had fallen asleep, but Mike hadn't closed his eyes yet.

In the morning, Mike woke her at 8 a.m. so she could get cleaned up, and get to Shoshone for her 9:00 a.m. doctor's appointment. No human ever looked so ghostly as Mike did after being up all night.

Cindy, on the other hand, was elated! "I was alive, and felt good! I drank more clay water on rising this morning, and after removing the clay rig I cleaned up and felt really great. I must say though, the stocking was gross."

The clay had absorbed a remarkable amount of toxic substances.

The Doc, a PA (Physician's Assistant), was a decent man, but was rather odd at times. People all over the area were talking about the incredible effects of Clay Therapy, and he went absolutely ballistic at the merest mention of our clay.

He told people, "That stuff will turn to rock in your system."

None of his clients dared tell him that they were using my clay. God forbid!

Cindy's appearance at the clinic that morning stunned the doc and his nurses. They couldn't believe that she looked and acted so well. This same man had made the asinine remark that, "You'll be lucky to be alive in twenty-four hours." Here she was twenty-four hours later, enjoying herself.

"Come in, please," said the Doc, motioning her inside to the examination room, and said in a very analytical fashion, "Let's re-examine this situation." After a few minutes he said, "We know that Valley Hospital confirmed that she had Toxic Shock Syndrome, right? She had all the symptoms, right?"

The nurse interjected, "Doctor, you thought she might not live twenty four hours."

He stared at his nurse in disbelief.

"You said that yesterday."

"I know what I said yesterday, thank you!" He began to read from his case history. "Did she have these symptoms, or not?" He read on, "Did she have lesions, or not?"

"She did have lesions," the nurse said.

"Then where are they now? Do you see any lesions now?"

"No, Doctor. There are no lesions present now."

"Then where did they go?"

"I don't know, Doctor!" the nurse replied.

This was becoming a comedy routine, and Cindy was enjoying every second of it. This physician had made a heartless although possibly accurate remark twenty-four hours earlier, and now had been made to look like a fool! On the other hand, this was a good man, doing his best to be an effective physician. Who wouldn't have responded the same way? Her recovery didn't make sense.

As she and Mike made ready to leave, he asked, "Cindy, did you take all the antibiotics real quick?"

"No, I kept throwing them up."

"Can you account for anything that made you recover so quickly and completely?"

"You should have asked me earlier. Sure, I know why, but you never asked me that. It was Cano's stuff, inside and out all night!"

With that they were out the door, jumped into that old rattletrap truck, and waved goodbye.

Mike created more rigs for Cindy's healing process, and she took full body clay baths daily, drank clay water, and completed her recovery.

ଓ ଓ ଓ

Some people in the past viewed my affection for the clay as eccentric behavior. Those same good people, when exposed to her benefits in their own family's lives changed their point of view and became a simple dyed-in-the-wool Clay Disciple. Of course you can see why.

Chapter 24

The Injured Bunny

My feeling is that there is nothing in life but refraining from hurting others, and comforting those that are sad.

Olive Schreiner

Our hearts went out to her instantly. Withdrawn and pale, the small, frail blonde in her mid-forties, had straight, fine hair. Joyce called me at the Miners Diner and told me about the woman who had just arrived and that I should see her. I thought it unusual for her to call me at the café, but something in her tone alerted me.

I saw the woman before she saw me. I know of nothing sadder than a person in pain and frightened in the midst of happy people. When I walked onto our beautiful parachute-covered patio, I picked her out immediately.

When I was a boy, I killed a young rabbit and then was instantly filled with regret. The moment impressed me deeply with the fragility and sanctity of life, and never again would I take away the existence of an innocent animal. I watched this woman closely, and sensed a person similar to the bunny rabbit, which immediately sparked my protective feelings for that helpless creature.

When I walked up on the patio I greeted the guests gathered there, many of whom I hadn't seen for awhile. There was always a wonderful spirit of vitality and gratitude at the Crystal Cross.

Everyone connected with our Healing Center knew that we were jointly, staff and guests, involved in the ongoing process of creating and experiencing the first genuine pure Therapeutic Clay Center in the country. We knew who we were, where we were, why we were there and that our clay was the cause of it all. We took a confident approach to our lady's ability to heal.

Apparently, our new little bunny sensed this. I went directly to her and offered her my hand as she stood up from her chair. She bypassed my hand and put her arms around my shoulders. I held her until she broke the embrace. She was a bunny rabbit in search of a sanctuary.

I hadn't yet said a word, and neither had she. Her soft, aqua blue eyes spoke volumes to me of her pain at being so alone. Her name was Laura Wilson.

She said, "I understand that you folks enjoy helping people."

"I believe that's an accurate description of the common denominator here at the Crystal Cross which brings us all together."

She smiled. "My, but that's a long answer."

I laughed a bit and said, "It is, isn't it? It's just that here the givers are the receivers and the receivers are the givers. It wasn't planned, it just turned out that way. What have you got to give?"

We sat down and she cried in a way that made me feel that she had cried many times before.

As she described her situation I realized that I'd never heard of anything like it. I didn't know that this condition existed, but it apparently ruled her daily existence. She was ultra-sensitive, and was in fact allergic to a variety of things, an incredible number of substances that we encounter in every day life. Her illness, which I predict will become a veritable nightmare for millions more in the 21st century, grew into a major interest for me. She suffered from Multiple Chemical Sensitivity.

She didn't know how, or where it started. It could have been any little exposure to something that triggered the start of severe reactions to innumerable substances in the environment. She was extremely sensitive to the environment.

How I deeply resent the stupid and inhumane position of some physicians who contend that these reactions are a learned response!

She stayed with us about a month. We so much enjoyed working with her, and in return, she helped out taking care of other guests when she could. The detoxing clay baths were a godsend to her, and she was less stressed. It was inspiring to watch her improve. Then two situations occurred to break the spell.

She had a problem to deal with in the Midwest somewhere and we had started more construction. Saws were sawing, trucks were rolling around, the backhoe was digging, and the bulldozer was moving a lot of real estate. The very air she breathed became her enemy, and she had no way to avoid it.

We needed to physically isolate her, and we didn't yet have the facilities available for her needs. It was heartbreaking to see her cave in. We all sank a little bit as she left for Missouri, and many in our community gathered to let her know that we'd be ready for her to return when the construction was finished. She could have a home with clean air, clean healing water and Therapeutic Clay.

However, things didn't work out as we'd hoped. Our little bunny committed suicide in Springfield on New Year's Day 1992.

Give me health and a day, and I will make the pomp of emperors ridiculous.   Ralph Waldo Emerson

Chapter 25

Hot Times On Cajón Pass

You can do anything in this world if you're prepared to take the consequences.   W. Somerset Maugham

Coming out of Los Angeles, California on I-15, a stretch of 20 miles or so pulls one up out of the Los Angeles Basin and into the high desert. Thousands of travelers have met their Waterloo about five miles into that magnificent Cajón Pass. Nowhere else in the entire United States will a traveler encounter a more brutal test for a vehicle's engine and cooling system. If you have a weak system this steep grade will get you quick. It's notorious.

One hot August Friday in 1989, I drove along the packed freeway. At 5:00 p.m., the mercury still hovered in the high 90s. My heavy-duty crew cab pickup truck was outfitted with everything necessary for handling any problem or emergency, and I certainly always carried extra one-gallon containers of bottled water. On more than one occasion I helped out a traveler new to the desert with my water.

On this particular day, I followed directly behind a ten-year old camping rig starting up Cajón Pass. Early into the long pull to the top, it was clear the truck was struggling. It's amazing how many people continue up that hill, even with their engine overheating, gambling that they can force their vehicle to the top without serious damage.

There! He began to hug the right shoulder and slowed down. Steam spewed from under the hood. I slowed and stopped when he did, pulling right behind him. Usually by pouring water on the hot, but running radiator, letting it cool some, and then getting the hot cap off, I could then fill the radiator, and get the individual back on the road.

But something didn't feel right to me. The driver didn't look like he belonged in an old, seasoned camper. He looked like a city guy who probably hadn't camped out since he was a boy. He looked like he had taken to the road in someone else's camper.

He wore a Coors beer shirt, shorts and thongs. He could have been the poster boy for the Get Away Day. When he got out of the rig with a bath towel in his hands, I was already walking toward him.

"Looks like she's hot!"

"Yes, she was fine a few minutes ago, then, well, there it is."

"I can understand. It happens fast this time of day. Can I give you a hand? I have water."

"You do?" He looked so relieved.

"Let me get it. Be right back."

He lifted the hood. The radiator was going wild. I had two gallons of water, and was almost back to the front of the truck when I saw a bad mistake in progress. He had the towel folded a couple of times, and had it over the spewing radiator. Before I could say or do anything he began to twist and force the cap, a very dangerous move.

Then it blew!

For a microsecond he tried to control the steam with the towel. Only his sunglasses kept the steam from directly hitting his eyes. He didn't instantly react and jump back out of the way. He held on for just a split second, but that was the worst mistake he could have made. The steam really nailed him.

I supported him for a moment. His wife came around from her

side of the truck and saw that he had been hit hard. By this time some other cars had pulled over to lend assistance. I ran to my toolbox where I had six one-gallon containers of gelled clay and tore the top off one. When I returned, I found him on the ground and obviously in a great deal of pain. His frightened wife knelt beside him as a crowd gathered.

I had never seen steam do that kind of damage. As I squatted beside him, I hesitated to act.

Then someone yelled, "Put some butter on him!"

That did it! Butter my ass! Why am I holding back? I'd told a lot of people about various injuries to get it on quick. So, do it! Do it now, Cano, and do it complete. And I damn well did just that.

Thank God I had a full gallon of gelled clay rather than just little plastic tubs that I used for samples.

His glasses were already off so I covered his entire face and ears with clay then spread it over his entire neck and chest. With God as my witness, before I finished his arms he was mumbling about how cool and good it felt on his face.

"My God, what is that stuff?" He couldn't believe it.

After a few minutes he was resting on the ground.

The people in the crowd were asking, "What's that stuff on his face and arms?"

I pulled his wife aside. "Ma'am, the EMTs will be here soon. I know what I'm doing and I did what I thought was best."

"Yes, and thanks. What is that stuff? I mean, he calmed down real quick and seems to have so much less pain."

"This is a natural solution of trace minerals. I can tell you more about it later. For now, though there's something I want to suggest. When the EMTs get here, they'll probably want to take the solution off because they don't know what it is. For sure they'll remove it when they get him to the hospital. That will be a big mistake, but that's your choice. He's been burned, but it's not critical. No matter though, this stuff is incredible for treating any kind of burn."

Very calmly she asked, "What's your name?"

"Graham, Cano Graham. I own a Therapeutic Clay Center up in the desert by Death Valley. That's why I know about this."

"This is clay? Like C-L-A-Y?"

I nodded.

"I'm going with a hunch, because I can see him resting. I believe you're right on."

I felt a lot better, "Thanks so much."

"Thank you! What will they do if we won't go to the hospital?"

"Well, first off they'll think you're nuts. Then they'll examine him and see that he's not in too much pain and no doubt help you get him in the truck."

"What else do I need to know?"

"I'll get to that in a second. But first, will you have any trouble driving back?"

"No, that's not a problem. He won't have any problem sitting there for half an hour, will he?"

"No, the steam just hit him on the neck, arms, face and a little on the chest. I think that he'll be able to walk and sit with very little problem."

"That's good. Now, what do I do when we get home?"

"Just a second and I'll tell you. First I'll get the radiator filled. There's a turnaround not a half-mile up the freeway, so you'll be going back down the hill soon. You say your home is just a half-hour away?"

"Yes, we live in Covina."

"Oh sure, I know it well. Now then, by the time you get home, this will be almost dry. Soak it off with wet, warm towels, and reapply all over the burn area. If it's a little hard to get off, don't worry about it. Just spread the clay over the part that won't come off easily, no problem. In a couple of days just use a thick, watery solution over the burned area. Keep reapplying, soaking and reapplying. You'll both see an amazing healing process. Mrs., excuse me, I don't know your name!"

"We're the Hicks from Covina. He's George and I'm Wendy."

"Well, Mrs. Hicks, it's nice to meet you. You're a brave soul to take all of this so calmly."

"I'm falling to pieces inside."

"Now, you're doing fine. By the way, I'm going to get you enough clay to last you through the entire healing process."

"How long will it take?"

"You'll see results soon, real soon. A month from now he'll be brand new. George shouldn't develop any infection, and within a few days you'll really start noticing the results. Just keep applying and soaking, and use a good Aloe Vera cream as a moisturizer later in the healing process."

She started to thank me.

I stopped her. "Mrs. Hicks, I know how you feel. I really do. I appreciate your response, but it's completely unnecessary."

I had to get things done and get out of there. I went back to my truck and grabbed a couple of gallon size containers, along with some of the dry powder.

I explained what I was doing and put the containers in her truck. I handed her my card from the Crystal Cross Therapeutic Clay Center.

"Okay, this ought to do it. This will easily last you until he's completely healed. Keep using it until all the new skin has grown back. Also, Mrs. Hicks, have him drink the clay water twice a day. The instructions are on the label."

"You drink it too?"

"Yep, sure do…in fact it is very important that you both take it internally!"

"But I wasn't burned."

"No, but you were hit emotionally, and you've got a lot to go through."

I took another look at George and found him resting easily. He trusted his wife to do the right thing. He looked up at me and said,

"Man, thanks a lot. If I can ever..."

I broke in and said, "Mrs. Hicks has my card. Come up and see me when you get squared away."

They replied in unison, "We sure will!"

I asked, "What kind of work do you do?"

"I'm a salesman for a paper company, and Wendy is a schoolteacher in San Dimas."

Mrs. Hicks wrote down their address and handed it to me.

ೞ   ೞ   ೞ

They became regulars at my place. You should have heard George tell the story of this guy smearing clay all over him. We've had some good times since that day. He loves to stick his chin out and say, "See! No scars!"

Chapter 26

Potato—Potato—Potato

Men imagine that they can communicate their virtue or vice only by overt actions. And do not see that virtue or vice emit a breath every moment.   Ralph Waldo Emerson

In the desert an eyeball hot day means just what it implies: when the heat reaches a certain zone, even your eyeballs get hot. And a real scorcher produces another phenomena: the air seems to vibrate. It's true; a low hum without apparent source thickens the air. The late afternoon of July 6, 1989 had been an eyeball hot, humming day.

I'd been on the road for three hours in a truck that had no air conditioning. I was almost home, but I needed a break. For the past half-hour I'd been visualizing a double Bailey's over ice for starters, followed by a big ham steak and eggs. Pike's Restaurant in Baker, California knew how to treat a hot, tired traveler, and I was a regular.

Ah, relief! The restaurant booth felt cool to the touch. Doris, a pure fan of the Crystal Cross, and my favorite waitress, saw me drive up.

She had the ice water waiting and said, "Hi, Cano. The same?"

"Hi, gal. Yes, thanks. And have Ed do the eggs basted, and wheat toast."

"You got it. What's new at the Cross?"

"We're getting her done. Just built a new hot tub. By the way, there's some evil looking storm clouds southwest of here. I just missed 'em, but they're heading this way. Thought you might want to tell your kids."

"Yes, thanks, a trucker just told me about it. We need a good rain."

I wolfed down the water. Doris quickly refilled it, set my Bailey's down and smiled at our routine. Just as I was about to take a sip of my favorite drink on Earth, a playful six-year-old popped her head over the booth in front of me. She wanted my attention.

I winked twice, and she winked in return. Our communication was confirmed.

Her grandmother smiled at me and said, "Stop bothering that man."

I assured the grandmother that the little one was no trouble at all, and that in fact I enjoyed her, and thought that we were friends. I stole a glance at the little one, and as if on cue, she nodded vigorously in agreement. The grandmother understood, and with charming alacrity asked me to join the family, so they could better get to know the little one's new-found friend. I accepted the offer, and before long we were talking, and getting acquainted.

The family, the Bradshaws from El Monte, California, were returning from Las Vegas. The family consisted of the grandmother, her son and daughter-in-law and their little girl. The grandmother and little one were traveling in a van while the son and daughter-in-law accompanied them, riding a Harley-Davidson motorcycle.

I remember my first impression of the son, Stoney, and how much he resembled his mother. They resembled each other in their eyes, speech, and in a certain presence I sensed in each of them.

Stoney, a big man, owned a motorcycle shop. His leather cap, boots and chaps only added to the impression of a no nonsense type of guy. But as soon as he began to talk, I understood that his appearance belied a keen mind and the heart of one with a love of life, and respect for humanity.

His wife, Valerie, was a striking girl; tall and slim with dyed black hair and matching eyes. I learned she was a dancer, but didn't ask what kind of dancer.

Through the introductions and conversation, the wheels in my head kept turning. And when the family asked about me, I did not break my pattern, but talked about the Crystal Cross Clay Center.

I explained to Stoney that mechanics, for example, who always bang their hands and fingers, had found it a good idea to keep a supply of gelled and dry clay on hand. I told him I knew for a fact that many bike riders in Las Vegas carried clay with them in case of an emergency, whether for cuts or burns, either for themselves or others.

Then Stoney made my day. "Cano, how does the clay work on arthritis?"

"Are you kidding? That's one of the main uses. Do you know someone with arthritis?"

Stoney paused, and then the Grandmother, Peggy said, "It's me, we've just been talking about it. I have a very painful arthritic knee. Do you really think it would help?"

"Do I? Don't go anywhere. I'll be right back." As I left the booth I asked, "Does it hurt now?"

"It's driving me wild. And all the traveling doesn't help, either." She unconsciously rubbed her left knee.

"This won't take but a few seconds." I went to my truck, got a jar of gelled clay and returned. I could see their curiosity.

"Left knee?" I inquired.

And then in unison I heard, "Now? Here?"

"Does it still hurt?" I smiled like we were playing a game.

"Yes!" she said.

I winked at the little one and asked, "What's your name?"

That made her happy. Grinning in a cute way she cooed, "Allison."

213

"Okay then, why don't we have their dessert special, some more coffee, and let me show you what this stuff can do in half an hour?" They couldn't resist my offer.

I asked Peggy to raise her dress above the knee. We shared a laugh, and then I spread the clay over, around and behind the knee. I unfolded some paper napkins to cover the clay, making it less messy so she could lower her dress. Allison scooted under the table and sat beside me. We were solid friends by now. Then, we enjoyed our hot apple pie and ice cream and began to talk.

No more than five minutes had passed, when the violent wind and rainstorm I'd seen began tearing through the area. We had front row seats for the sudden fury swirling directly in front of the restaurant.

The whole scene brought a certain intimacy to our group. For forty-five minutes we shared a happy rapport, completely forgetting where we had been, where we were going, or about the clay.

Peggy needed to stretch, stood up slowly and exclaimed, "Dear God in Heaven! I can't believe it! Mr. Graham, it's happened to me! Oh, dear Lord! It's real! Oh kids, the pain just left me*!"* She flexed her left knee out into the aisle, up and down, up and down.

"Mom, I can't believe it!" Stoney pounded the booth for added emphasis. Peggy fell into the booth next to her son and began crying on his shoulder. He was laughing, and had his arm around her.

She began laughing, and kicking her leg like a schoolgirl. She said, "Kids, this is too much!" Then Peggy became more subdued, and added, "This kind of thing never happens to me, it always happens to someone else."

By this time the manager had come over to see what all the excitement was about. I knew the manager. She and her boyfriend often came to the Cross for a stress down as she called it. "What's up, Cano?"

"Well, I found a real good arthritic knee."

Marge nodded and smiled. "And you put your clay on the knee?"

"Sure did."

Allison, standing on the booth next to me, said to the manager, "Mr. Graham made my granny's knee hurt more better. He did!"

The manager picked Allison up, hugged her, and said, "I know just how Granny feels. Look at this." She started flexing her fingers. "Do you remember what I was going through Cano?"

"Sure do, Marge. Have you had any more trouble with that hand?"

"Every now and then. But not at all like it was, and even then I just slap some clay on it, and that's all she wrote."

Turning to Peggy, she said, "I really do know how you feel. It's unbelievable, isn't it?"

I asked Marge to have the busboy bring some hot, damp towels and soaked off what remained. From my experience I knew just how good this felt to Peggy. Then the storm passed, which seemed appropriate. Like many desert storms, it had surprising strength but was short lived. Meeting the Bradshaw's, sharing a meal, and giving them a little clay demonstration, well, the story seemed complete. But, little did I know that it had another chapter to go.

We exchanged addresses, and said goodbye. What a great family. I thought, how fortunate they are to have each other. I watched Peggy and her granddaughter hop in the van, while her son toweled off his Harley. As I turned to Marge, I heard Stoney start the bike.

"Bloom! Potato...potato...potato...potato."

(If you say it fast enough, Potato-potato-potato-potato is the sound of a Harley-Davidson at idle, or moving along at slow throttle.)

I turned back and saw Peggy and Allison wave from the van, and then start off to the highway, heading west.

And then, I experienced a nightmare in slow motion.

Stoney and his lady had just gotten their things adjusted on the bike, and turned to their right to wave at me and Marge. They couldn't see the pickup truck entering the lot behind them from the left. The truck moved fast.

I saw it all in grinding slow motion and yelled, "Nooooooo!"

Stoney and his lady turned back to the front and started to pull out just as the truck hit them. It must have been going at least 30 miles per hour, and knocked them a good thirty feet, and the bike fifty feet. The truck careened by, barely missed running over them, and stopped only after it crashed into a big Ryder rental truck parked at the side of the road.

I sprinted toward them thinking my God, they're both dead. Neither of them moved. I soon saw that Valerie, though conscious, was not moving, and Stoney was in bad shape. I was scared.

Stoney had severe, deep lacerations on his face, and a truly ugly wound on his left shoulder and rib cage. Blood gushed.

Marge ran out of the restaurant toward us. "Cano, I called 911 but the EMTs are already responding to an emergency on the east side of town. They won't get here for fifteen or twenty minutes."

As a young kid, I served as a Paratrooper in Korea. It had been that long since I saw that much blood and such serious injury. I knew that I had to try and stop the bleeding.

I scrambled to my truck, grabbed a towel and some dry, powdered clay. I tore Stoney's shirt open, soaked up what blood I could from the lacerations, and poured dry powder directly into his wounds. In fact, I spread the cuts open with my fingers and pour the clay directly into the gaping cuts. I'd done this on minor cuts, and had once done it on a dog that had been sliced wide open, but never on a human injured like this.

Then, out of the crowd in back of me came a voice, "What in God's name are you doing, man?"

I assumed he was talking to me, and without looking up I said, "I'm trying to stop the bleeding! What the hell do you think I'm doing?"

The voice replied, "Sir, I'm a dentist from Newport Beach, California, and I'm telling you that you could be sued for everything you own for doing what you're doing."

All I could say was, "Get him the hell away from me!"

Very quickly, the blood gushing out of the wounds slowed. The whole thing was messy as hell, but the busboy brought water and some fresh towels, and I continued to wipe the blood away, looking to isolate the deeper problems, and see if any arteries were severed. He was lucky. The left shoulder was raw meat. His upper body trembled from the trauma. He was barely conscious, and close to shock. Someone from the crowd covered him with a blanket. The mixture of blood and clay covered the left side of his face.

I told him, "Valerie is shook-up, but otherwise okay, and your mom is right here, Stoney. Your daughter, too."

Peggy said, "Hi, dear. I looked back when I didn't see you following, but we must have driven five miles farther before we could turn around." Then, with the sight of so much blood and the evident pain her son was in, she turned away and grabbed my shoulder to steady herself.

I tried to console her. "Peggy, most of the bleeding has slowed or stopped, and he appears stable."

We needed a doctor. I knew that Stoney's leg was broken, but it wasn't a life threatening injury. However, the possibility of internal injuries bothered me. I asked someone to get the dentist. He was standing behind me, and bent down close. I asked him if he thought Stoney had any internal injuries. He said he couldn't be sure, but he didn't think so because Stoney wasn't bleeding from the mouth.

Then the dentist squatted down beside me and said, "This has been very interesting."

"Interesting?" I replied, shaking my head. Doctors always seem to choose the word *interesting* for the results of clay therapy.

He asked, "This is clay therapy? What's in the stuff that stops bleeding so quickly?"

"If I told you, you wouldn't believe me. Just trace minerals, the stuff you're made of. Seriously, it's a special type of clay."

About that time, the EMTs pulled into the parking lot, twenty-five minutes after the truck had smashed into Stoney and Valerie.

As one of them sized up the scene, one of the EMTs saw the mess on Stoney, and gasped, "What the hell? What's this stuff? Did it stop the bleeding?"

His partners knew me, and recognized the clay. He was about to explain when Peggy stepped beside me, grasped my right hand, and smiled, "It's God's clay, the stuff you're made of."

Allison still frightened and crying, held tightly to her grandmother.

As they loaded Stoney and Valerie into the ambulance, Peggy, Allison, and I approached the stretchers. We assured them both that we'd see them in an hour or so at the hospital in Barstow. Stoney mumbled something about his bike. I told him that I'd take it to his shop in El Monte. We watched the ambulance pull away. Peggy and Allison were very brave.

ឥ   ឥ   ឥ

Several months later on Thanksgiving Day reservations had been confirmed with a large deposit to fully book the Crystal Cross for a special four-day retreat of some sort. But by noon, none of the guests had arrived and I was a bit pissed off. I really thought the whole affair, whatever it was, might be a no show. Then down the road, I saw a van coming with its horn honking, and a little blonde girl who looked like Allison waved wildly out the window. A dozen Harley Davidson motorcycles followed closely behind. What an entrance!

Potato…potato…potato…in concert. They sounded like a huge, distant chorus of rolling thunder.

My neighbors came outside to watch the slow-moving procession of bikers, and wondered if I knew what was happening. I caught on quickly when I saw Peggy and Allison in their van followed by Stoney and Valerie on their bike, and a host of Clay Disciples following. They had come prepared for their four-day party.

And party we did! Hot tubs, swimming in warm mineral water, and clay baths, good music and refreshments!

A few years later, Valerie gave birth to a little boy who looks just like Stoney. Peggy's knee is doing real well, and Allison has grown into a lovely young woman. I can hardly wait to see them again, or hear another refrain of potato… potato…potato…

Chapter 27

Curt The Streaker

The great end of life is not knowledge but action.

Thomas Huxley

My brother, Dr. Frank Graham, and his wife Jean had taken the day off to experience the clay baths. We were all about to enjoy a hot tub when Rick came running and yelling, "Cano, Curt has hurt himself!"

I instantly motioned to Frank and his friends to follow Rick.

"Damn it! Damn it!" My heart pounded.

Although the guys considered Curt a firm taskmaster, he sometimes became over-protective of the local inexperienced workers. Today, the third day of our Granddaddy construction, he grew impatient watching two young workers trying to maneuver a creosote soaked telephone pole into a hole. He was concerned they were going to make a serious mistake and get hurt. In a knee-jerk reaction to their situation, he jumped off the backhoe, brushed them aside, and grabbed the hot pole. Curt was already soaking wet with sweat, so even with his strength, it took some time to single handedly muscle the big slippery toxic pole into place.

The hot creosote quickly penetrated through his wet clothing soaking his arms, chest and legs with the volatile chemical. In a matter of seconds, the creosote began to cook his flesh.

When we got close, Dr. Frank said, "Oh, hell, Bud I believe he's hurt!"

None of us had ever imagined the big guy in pain, yet there he stood, helpless and trembling in distress, while frantically trying to tear his shirt off. His legs were soaked in front, and he began to have a serious reaction. Curt peeled out of his jeans, leaving only his shorts and cap, but the creosote continued to burn his upper legs and stomach.

Dr. Frank said, "Bud, I think he's almost in shock. Someone should call the EMTs and alert the closest hospital. I believe this man is in real trouble."

I said, "Damn it to hell! I don't think there's time!"

"Bud, it'll take *too* long."

"Son of a ... Curt! Lose the shorts and get into the clay pool."

Still trembling and stunned, Curt stammered, "Well ..."

"Come on, man, don't think about it. Just do it. Quick! Curt, get out of them *now*. You can leave your cap on!"

I wasn't trying to be funny. It just kind of popped out. But mentioning his cap seemed to snap him out of his state. The workers laughed at the cap remark, and Curt even half cracked a smile, although we knew this scene was anything but comical. He shed his shorts and started running for the big clay pool.

The workers encouraged the big guy by shouting, "Go Curt Go!"

He moved fast. Taking long loping strides, he closed fast on the clay pool.

No one who witnessed Curt streaking, whiter butt on pale skin, with only his trusty cap on for cover, will ever forget the memorable moment. That event was the central topic of conversation many a night at the bar, especially when describing how with one heroic leap, cap flying off, he dove, as gracefully as any Olympic diver, head first into the clay pool.

We all ran to the edge, anxious about his condition, and found him wiping clay off his eyes, and smiling like an old bear eating sweet spring berries.

I asked him, "How ya doin' in there? You didn't burn anything completely off, did ya?"

He first adjusted his old cap back on his clay-covered head, and said, "Cano, I never seen nothing like it. I mean the whole thing was over instantly when the clay covered me. I don't feel a doggone thing right now. Nothing. It's amazing. Darndest thing I ever heard of."

We all loved to see him smiling when he said, as if he was avoiding work, "I'm not getting out of here for a while."

I said, "Fine, stay all afternoon. Care for a cold beer?"

"As a matter of fact a cold one would work!"

Rick broke everyone up when he exclaimed, "Curt, I can sell a hundred tickets at five dollars a pop if you'll run through the whole scene just one more time! Of course you've got to let me film it!"

Dr. Frank put his arm around my shoulder, shook his head, and said, "I can't believe it. For God's sake where's this stuff been?"

"We're hiding it from the AMA."

Jean said, "Ha! I believe it after what I just saw!" Then she turned to Curt. "Are you still okay? No pain?"

Curt said, "No ma'am, no nothing."

Dr. Frank said, "Bud, if we had taken the time to drive Curt to a clinic, or even treat him here, I mean with the best of treatments, for the way he was hit, well, he'd be in a world of trouble, and could be in serious condition. I know this creosote will eat you up!" Frank turned to Rick. "Hell of a deal. Emergency Medicine should know about this!" Then to Curt he said, "Curt, I'm going to be here until later this afternoon. If you ever decide to come out of there, I'd like to confirm the condition of where you were burned."

Curt said, "No problem. I'll be out of here in a few minutes, then I'm gonna 'bake out.' I'll be around."

Frank put his arm around me and said, "Big Bro, I think you've found what you're supposed to do. You've got a different type of natural healing facility on your hands. I guess Herbert wasn't your last case."

"Herbert?" I didn't get it.

Bud smiled and said, "Yeah, Herbert, that old three-legged cat you brought home, remember? You slept with that creature."

Chapter 28

A Shoot

Men, like peaches and pears, grow sweet a little while before they begin to decay.   Oliver Wendell Holmes

We had an unusual day on our hands; windy, misty, and cold. The weather had been bad for a week, and I was sick of it. We had no calls for information, and only a few reservations. I saw no break in the weather forecast. I told Curt and the crew to take a few days off. I had one girl, Margarita, on duty, and a maintenance man hiding somewhere.

I looked out the window to check the weather, and saw a new suburban van coming up the road. I glanced a second time when I noticed a guy hanging out the window apparently filming the area as they drove in. His enthusiasm on such a nasty day was enviable. I also thought he was goofy.

I wasn't all that excited about dealing with customers or answering questions. I felt like the weather looked.

When the big van pulled in close I said out loud to myself, "Ye gods!" This looks like a vanload of smiling Japanese teenagers! I mumbled, "Give me a break!" Now I knew just how the ugly American felt.

Only one passenger exited the vehicle, a tall Japanese woman with short hair, black horned rimmed glasses, wearing a long expensive looking coat with a fur of some kind around the collar. Even from a distance she looked all business.

Grudgingly, I opened the door and stepped outside into a cold wet wind to meet her as I continued to mumble. I didn't realize they made tall women in Japan. The eager-eyed young people in the van were cute enough, waving and smiling like they had found an old friend. Friend or no friend they stayed in their van, either because they were told to, or because it was too cold to get out. Fine and dandy with me because I didn't care to mess with them.

As she approached the front steps I was suddenly thankful for the misty cold weather. If the weather had to be bad, so be it, and to add some strength to my position, I quickly prayed that the heavens would cause the day to get even worse so as to deter any other fools from bothering me.

I seemed to be praying a lot today, but regardless I didn't think a little more could hurt, "Dear Lord, let them just want directions to someplace else, anyplace, but not here!" Now I felt fully armed spiritually to meet this Asian intrusion.

When she stepped onto the porch, she stood relatively close to me, paused for a moment, and looked me directly in the eyes. She took my breath away. This slim, five-foot-nine-inch, shorthaired, fur-wearing businessperson was one beautiful woman. I pegged her at about 35-40 years old.

I blinked, cleared my throat, and said, "*Konnichi wa.*"

Unbelievable! I hadn't said, "Hello" in Japanese in over 35 years! I motioned to the door very gallantly and said, "Won't you come in, it's cold out here."

"Oh, *Konnichi wa.*" She drew the fur collar up around her neck and accepted my welcome by bowing slightly and thanking me. "*Kekko desu.* Yes, it is chilly outside."

What a difference a moment makes in one's view of the world. I must have appeared remarkably similar to the desk clerk at the Ambassador when trying to be hip, slick and cool as possible. "How can I help you? Please let me take your coat, and do make yourself comfortable."

She slid gracefully into a chair, crossed her legs, and purred, "You speak Japanese?"

"No, no, just hello, goodbye, thank you. I learned it while on R&R in Japan during the Korean War." I smiled at my own thought when I said, "About the time you were born."

"Oh, I see, but you still remember? Well, thanks again." She glanced around the room and nodded. "My it is cozy in here."

I responded, "Kekko desu. You know I love saying 'thank you' in Japanese."

"Good. I like to hear it too." She composed herself, became more serious and said, "Sir, the reason I'm in the area is because my company has been retained to find a suitable location for a Photo Shoot." She pointed out the window. "As you can see, I have some excited models who need a place to work for a day." She started fishing around in her coin purse."

"I understand." I wished the weather were a whole lot warmer. And can you believe those eyes?

She found what she was after, handed me her card, and smiled, "My name is Kuniko Hayashi and you are'?"

Whew! Do some women get prettier on cold days? "Ah, excuse me? Yes, uh, my name is Cano Graham. I own this place." I felt as though I'd answered a complex question. Her voice tasted like honey and her lips reminded me of little rosebuds. I'm nuts about roses anyway. Was I being obvious? She was just so darn good looking.

Kuniko said, "Actually, you've been recommended because of what you have here."

"*Kekko desu.* And who referred us may I ask?"

"It's a kind of round about introduction that started when a young Japanese family stopped by here almost a month ago. They said you toured them around your place during the noon hour."

"Yes, I remember they had a little boy and, and she had a blister from walking in Death Valley."

"That's it. Anyway, they told an uncle of mine who owns a restaurant in Las Vegas, and it all sounded interesting, the way they described it to him."

"Hmmm, strange how things work!" I was considering her explanation on one side of my brain, and how pretty she was on the other.

She continued. "I understand you have clay baths? And we can really get in them? Your whole body?"

"Sure, and it's a wonderful experience too."

"And hot mineral water tubs? A swimming pool that is covered? Does the pool have mineral water also?"

"Yep! We have all those things. What your uncle told you is true. But you'll see all that soon, Miss Hayashi."

She laughed, raised her right forefinger and said, "Plus the family said you were friendly."

I thought, oh, God lady, you have no idea just how friendly I feel right now! But instead, in a casual, ultra humble manner, I offered. "Oh, we enjoy making everyone comfortable."

"Mr. Graham, understand that…"

I couldn't bear to hear her use such formalities. "Please, call me Cano."

"Certainly, thanks. Cano? I like that name."

She was so cute!

"Anyway, as I was saying, *Cano*, please understand, naturally we pay a fee for using your place and you will certainly receive the proper credit wherever the stills and video are used."

"You mean today?"

She removed her glasses. "Yes, today. And we'd like to remain here most of the afternoon."

"But it's so cold and damp, and it will be that way all day."

She pointed to the Suburban and like a mother hen, said, "These kids don't mind. They're young models from Japan and want to work. They're game if you're willing."

"All afternoon? Well, outside in the clay baths will be chilly, but smearing it all over themselves inside the solarium will make some good pictures. And of course the hot tubs and swimming pool will be inside, so sure, I'm glad you came here. I'm sure it will be a creative shoot. If they can take the weather, I'll certainly do my best to make them comfortable and welcome."

"Thanks, we won't be any trouble."

"Kuniko, I'm curious, you're not from Japan?'

"No, no I'm a Californian all the way. Been in LA all my life. Went to USC, modeled for a few years, opened a travel agency, then started doing this for companies in Japan, and here I am."

"Yes, here we are, or rather here you are. Let me show you where you can dress, sorry, I mean *they* can dress. I'll have Margarita make a big pot of hot chocolate and get some towels for them. Do they have robes?"

"Yes, they do. And Cano, that is very thoughtful, really! Thank you, *kekko desu*."

"De nada, as my Spanish-speaking friends say. It's nothing. Just part of the deal. Come on, is it Miss or Missus?"

She looked over her glasses and said, "Miss," and smiled.

"Okay, let's get the show started." I suggested they shoot all the clay shots first. From there they could clean up and prepare themselves for the swimming pool shots, followed by a truly relaxing time in the hot tubs.

I knew the girls would be in awe of Margarita, noticeably part Indian, very pretty, and just by her nature a perfect 'Indian' hostess for the young models a long way from home.

When we stepped out on the porch, Kuniko motioned for the girls to come with her. They left the vehicle smiling, waving, and bowing as if they had landed at LA International Airport with the network news waiting.

I led them into our recreation room that had a nice fire going with incense burning as usual this time of year. Kuniko explained to the group that I had agreed to have them for the day, and went on to acquaint the group with the services at the Crystal Cross. I let the girls and the young soundman enjoy the fire, while I took Kuniko and the older cameraman to the dressing room and gave them a tour of what they could use to set up the shots.

The cameraman, a comical chubby man of about fifty, with unusually long hair, was more interested in my collection of boulders, and wanted to bundle the girls up and shoot on our boulders as well. I agreed that idea could make for a very different type shot. The exotic images of the boulders alone would create a powerful impression. All in all, I had some artists on my hands. There was a definite disciplined and professional demeanor about the group.

I let Kuniko and the cameraman discuss their plans while I darted inside to call Ruthie. "Hi gal, you ought to come over, there's a Japanese film crew here shooting some models. They're a pleasant group of people. You ought to come over here and watch them work."

Ruthie said, "In weather like this? I can't believe it. What's it for?"

"I'm not sure. They haven't said yet. Maybe a magazine or something."

"Hmmm, magazine possibly, huh?" Ruthie was interested in anything that would spread the word about what we were doing. "How much longer will they be there?"

"At least a couple of hours, maybe more. Why don't you pick up Sylvia and bring her along? She'd get a kick out of the way they'll work. They appear to be professional about the shoot."

"Be right over, does sound like fun."

"Also, Ruthie, the guide for the group wants to know where to eat? Who's cooking at the Miners Diner today?"

Ruthie brightened. She saw an opening. "They're hungry?"

"Yeah, I think so. If not, they soon will be. You know, they're working and it's miserable and all. Yeah, I think so. I had Margarita fix some hot chocolate, but there's not much else around here. Joyce has been in L.A. for a week."

"I'll pick up Sylvia, and be over in a few minutes. I've got to go to the store first."

The girls, like brave little troopers, smiled and posed in the crisp wind as if it were 90 degrees. Sylvia and Ruthie took a fast look at the bunch, threw up their hands, and retreated to the kitchen.

After the girls had worked in the clay pools and solarium, they washed up and shot in the hot tubs. The cameraman then decided to take a break to allow them to change swimsuits and redo their make up and hair for the swimming pool layout. As they got out of the hot tub, I suggested the girls throw on robes and come to the warm recreation room for some hot tea.

The suggestions surprised the crew and the models, but they thoroughly appreciated the invitation and the warmth of the fireplace.

Sylvia and Ruthie provided a huge punchbowl of piping hot split pea soup, and another bowl of those good kind of wheat crackers along with a nice salad, topped off with a slice of the famous date bread from Death Valley. We finished the meal in great spirits, and the girls had recharged their batteries for the pool work. Kuniko and the soundman went to their vehicle for a suitcase of swimsuits and a makeup chest.

Just then, the sound of Kuniko yelling in distress startled us.

The soundman yelled for help in Japanese, "*Tasuke! Tasuke! Tasuke!*"

I couldn't understand the words, but the tone of his voice indicated certain trouble. We all scrambled out the door to see Kuniko down on the ground and squirming in pain. She had stepped out of the Suburban, snagged the suitcase on something, stumbled and fell.

A quick look made me think she had broken her ankle. Through the tears she tried to stand but couldn't put any weight on the foot. I got her shoe off, and asked Sylvia to check the medicine cabinet for some of Joyce's back pain medication. The cameraman and I carried her to the recreation room, and pulled up a stuffed chair close to the fire. Sylvia returned without the pain medication saying, "Joyce must have taken the pain medication with her."

"Would you like some aspirin, Kuniko?"

"No, can't tolerate the stuff," she answered with a grimace.

I left her side momentarily to grab a crock of gelled clay behind the counter.

She saw me coming at her with the ceramic crock and asked, "Cano, what are you going to do? I don't know if its broken or not."

"Either way, broken or strained or sprained, we have to do something now. You have options though. As I see it the chances are this is a bad sprain and not broken. I've read about sprains lately and this seems too sensitive and painful for a break. One thing for sure, if I don't do something quick, this will swell up big time, really quick. Would you like to go to town or have me treat it with what I do?"

"Don't they treat a sprain or swelling with ice?"

"Yes, and it's good, but our clay has some distinct advantages over ice. First, the ice should only be on for like fifteen minutes, and then taken off and reapplied. You can keep this on for hours. The clay helps the body heal the damaged tissue. Ice doesn't."

She moved her ankle and moaned with the pain. "At this point, I just want the pain to go away. Just do it."

I immediately set to work. "I'd bet dinner it's not broken, but a bad sprain. The clay will reduce the swelling that's already started. It should help the pain in a minute or two as well. You'll be back on your feet faster this way than any other. Of course, if it works the way I say, you'll owe me a dinner sometime, someplace in L.A. Deal?"

She stuck out her hand. "*Sono tori desu.* You have a deal."

I rolled up her slacks a little and applied two big handfuls generously from above her ankle to cover most of her foot. As long as she wasn't going to be moving around it would be perfect for her to stay in front of the fire and 'bake out' her ankle.

When the cameramen saw we had everything under control, they went ahead and did the swimming pool shots.

Sylvia and Ruthie had a great sixth sense. They cleared the table, took everything to the kitchen and cleaned up.

I propped Kuniko's foot up on a box so she could shift around and bake out both sides of her foot. "Do you need anything?"

"No, I'm fine. I can't believe it. You win! I owe you dinner!"

"Already? Come on, it's only been ten minutes."

"Seriously, I feel relief, no kidding. I hate pain. It's my foot and I feel real relief!"

"In that case, take me someplace to eat where they dance slow."

"Yes, I know just the place in Marina Del Rey."

As I stoked the fire and threw on a log I said, "My, my. Marina Del Rey. That's uptown for a country boy from Tecopa."

"You have quite a place here. You love it don't you?"

I pulled up a chair beside her. "Yes, Kuniko, I do. Someday, our community will be known all over the world for our clay therapy. People get help for all kinds of ailments, some of which you will see by tomorrow morning I might add."

She rested her head on a pillow as she adjusted her foot to the heat. "Thanks Cano, a lot."

ဢ   ဢ   ဢ

The shoot went well and everyone went away pleased with the experience. I learned later that only two weeks after the shoot, it was shown on the Japanese *Tonight Show* in Tokyo, Japan.

With that exposure, the land of the rising sun had effectively discovered the Crystal Cross Therapeutic Clay Center. It so happens that I hadn't heard the last of the Japanese in general or Kuniko in particular. She dances the same as her voice sounds.

Chapter 29

Matthew 10:26

Everyone becomes brave when he observes one who despairs.
Friedrich Wilhelm Nietzsche

Joyce and I went to Sonora, California, to visit her family, and it delighted me to find that they had all been busily spreading the word about the clay.

Joyce hung up the phone and said, "That's interesting. Clara says she has a friend with a skin disorder, a fungus she's had for eleven years."

"What kind of fungus?" I asked.

"Big blotches all over her body. In the last six months it's started to move closer to her neck."

I asked the name of the dermatitis.

"She didn't say, but she did mention that for the past eleven years she's gone to all sorts of dermatologists, and has taken every known treatment. She's spent a mountain of money, but gotten no relief."

"Good," I said.

"Cano! You shouldn't say that! Someone might overhear you and get the wrong idea! Poor thing. Can you imagine? Eleven years?"

"Great! Wonderful!"

"Cano, stop that! I mean, really."

I was putting her on, in my own way. "Joyce, it's like this. I hate destruction caused by forest fires and tornadoes, but if they're going to happen, I don't want to miss the show. I wanted to see 'em close up and personal. As long as she has this condition, and nothing has worked, then let's see if we can help!"

Joyce shook that beautiful head of hers, and smiled at my enthusiasm. She understood my sense of humor.

Joyce and I went to Laura and Carl's to see how we could help with Laura's fungus problem. From the looks of the big rig parked outside, her husband was a trucker who hauled lumber for a living. When he opened the door to their home, his 6'6", 300-pound frame filled the doorway. He appeared to be the absolute incarnation of a mountain man.

He wore a bathrobe that could have doubled for a king size bedspread. He was huge, with thinning, long copper colored hair, and a big, bushy red beard. I immediately became aware that something was wrong with him by the tentative way he moved, and I assumed that the robe covered the reason for his constrained movement.

In a soft, mellifluous voice he said, "Come in Mr. Graham, and you must be Joyce. I'm Carl Elkins, and my wife is Laura. She'll be right out. She's changing clothes. Please, have a seat and get comfortable."

We followed him in and took a seat.

"Would you care for some freshly brewed coffee?"

"Yes, thanks. It smells wonderful."

He went into the next room and returned with three steaming, cups of coffee. Carl politely waited until we had a sip of the fresh brew before continuing.

"Well, Mr. Graham, I understand that you have a unique place down in the Death Valley area?"

This man had an almost regal aura about him, and I assumed by the religious articles in the home that he was a devout person.

At least someone was. I sensed it was he, and that he lived by his faith daily.

"Yes, I do have a rather unusual place. We have hot mineral water and therapeutic clay pools."

"That's what we understand. Therapeutic Clay, huh?" He seemed interested. He offered us cream and sugar for our coffee, and uncovered a plate of home made rolls. "I think you'll enjoy these. Laura's a fine baker. Help yourself."

As we stirred our coffee, he said, "Do you know Mr. Graham, that clay is mentioned often in the Bible?"

I said, "Please Carl, call me Cano. Yes, people have pointed out that fact to me before. Of course, we know that Clay Therapy is very ancient, and was used fairly extensively even before the time of Jesus."

"That's what I've been told. However, Jesus certainly advanced the cause when he put it in the blind man's eyes." He smiled broadly, enjoying his own remark.

I said, "I know a lady who would sure like to meet you. Maybe someday, who knows?"

"Oh, who?"

"My mom."

He thought for a moment and asked, "Why?"

"Oh, I believe she'd like you both you, and especially your comment about Jesus putting clay in the blind man's eyes."

"Now I understand. Well I hope so. One day."

After one minute of conversation I knew I was in the presence of a very thoughtful, bright and interesting man. He made us both feel very comfortable.

When Laura came into the front room, Carl introduced us. He moved uneasily. We made small talk about some people we knew in town who used the clay for various reasons, but the conversation inevitably turned to exotic rashes and fungal infections, the reason for our visit.

"Laura, I'm very curious. I don't see any sign of blotches on your arms or face. You have it all on your upper body?"

She wore slacks, with a big beach towel covering a small halter-top. She threw off the towel exposing big blotches, three to four inches in diameter. They were all over her upper body, front and back, above the waist, up to her neck.

The sight fascinated me. "I don't understand a lot about fungus. Why just on the upper body, and not on the arms themselves?"

Laura sounded scared when she said, "They're moving toward my face."

I saw multicolored blotches, with newer blotches overlapping the older ones.

"Is it true that you've suffered from these for eleven years?"

She nodded and glanced at Carl. "Yes, eleven years and I've tried everything that the doctors prescribed. My dermatologist has done everything in his power to help. The drugs slow it up, but not for long. It's getting worse." She raised her chin, "I'm afraid that it's spreading to my face." The fungus had reached her neck.

Carl asked, "Cano, can you tell me more about the rashes and other skin problems you've worked with?"

"Well, the word has been spreading about just how effective our particular clay is for treating these things, and some of them are certainly unusual. People get some strange skin maladies. We've had our share of the usual garden-variety type of problems of eczema. Psoriasis is a tough one. We've had several cases that nothing would touch, until we tried the clay on them. The results were great.

"You have to keep on top of stuff, though. People stop using it because they think that they're all healed. Suddenly the infection comes back, but if they continue to use clay regularly, people can even control psoriasis. Probably the biggest win for us though is seeing the clay work on acne. It's really amazing! This clay kills the bacteria that causes acne, and helps the whole area get back to normal."

236

Then Carl said, "You haven't mentioned shingles."

That was it! The reason for the robe, and the uneasiness. Carl had shingles, plus his wife had bad fungal blotches, and nothing helped either of them.

I asked, "Carl, how long have you had the stuff?"

"Too long. Have you ever had shingles?"

"No," I replied.

"It's driving me crazy, and I'm driving Laura and the children nuts. I've always been pretty healthy. Never had anything I couldn't shake." He remembered something. "She didn't mention it, but Laura has an itching problem too."

"Okay, enough. I'll be right back." I went to my truck and brought a big cookie jar full of beautifully gelled clay, soft and smooth, just perfect. This was great. I had a full-blown case of shingles in front of me and knew that my lady was about to heal the problem quicker than the Lord can get the news.

"Joyce, you do Laura and I'll do Carl."

Joyce and Laura went into the bedroom as Carl gently removed the robe. Ouch! It hurt to look at the welts and oozing sores! It covered much of his right rib cage.

Carl raised his arm so that I could see better. What a mess.

Then he said, "I had it for a while before I ever tried to find an answer, and by that time nothing would help."

I knew a lot about the subject of shingles. I had read extensively about it, but hadn't seen but about a half dozen cases. Of those I'd seen, his was the worst. I began to apply a big handful of clay to the problem area.

"We've prayed about finding a healer. You just might be the one."

I drew back. "Let's get this straight Carl. I'm no healer. Clay Therapy has made a lot of very regular people look as if they were healers. A monkey could put it on, and it's not a big deal to get it off. I'm not a healer, I'm a Disciple, a Clay Disciple."

"Is that what you call yourself? A Clay Disciple? That's

great!" he exclaimed.

I applied the clay and said, "Okay, that does it. You'll probably feel some relief before too long."

"Is that it?"

"Yep, that's it! When it dries, soak it off with warm towels, and then repeat the process again and again, until it's completely gone." I looked up, and that big man had large tears running down his cheeks; such a gentle soul.

"Thank you Lord, and thank you, Mr. Graham."

That remark seemed a bit much, but I let it go. My lady was already taking the edge off the stinging pain. He said, "I can already *feel it*. Oh, I just want it to help Laura, too. I know it will! You mentioned that people have been using clay therapeutically for thousands of years?"

"Yes, my research tells me it's *at least* that old."

He wrapped his big hands around the Bible that lay on the mantle over the fireplace. Carl tilted his head back, crossed his hands, holding the Bible over his chest and asked, "Cano, you don't read the Bible much do you?"

"Sorry, no I don't."

He spoke with reverence in his voice saying, "There is nothing covered that shall not be revealed, and hidden that shall not be known." Then with a child-like radiance in his eyes he said, "Cano, that's Matthew 10:26."

Within thirty days, he and Laura enjoyed remarkable results. The shingles were long gone and fresh, pink skin covered the unsightly blotches on Laura.

Chapter 30

Thumbs Up Dog!

A large part of altruism, even when it's perfectly honest, is grounded upon the fact that it is uncomfortable to have unhappy people about one.   H. L. Mencken

What could be more fun than watching an Italian family host a special dinner party? Lou and Angela Caruso had placed the last dishes on the table. The wine and conversation flowed.

From across the recreation room, Lou raised his chubby hand in the air, signaled a thumbs up and yelled, "Hey Dog! Hey Baby! Let's get after it!"

Angela, Ruthie, Sylvia and Joyce, said, "It's ready, let's get it on."

I laughed along with my friends about Lou's streetwise language, and his way of doing things. I love to see people enjoy themselves, and Lou was completely beside himself.

I acknowledged Lou's request, and the dozen or so guests began to move toward their seats.

Lou's Robert DeNiro looks and his gregarious personality had already captured me a few months earlier, and had begun to entice my friends a few hours previously.

Then, in a scene similar to the one where the Italian boss stands up before a huge gathering to make an announcement of some kind, Lou started tapping his glass with a spoon. He wanted everyone's attention. He started off saying a few nice things about our place, what a pleasure it was being there and so forth, when he raised his glass for a final toast. I swear he reminded me of Robert DeNiro when he looked around the room. He waited for a serious moment then said, "I came to Vegas. I wanted to play. I lost my money, but found Cano's clay! Yeahhhhh!" And he thrust his hands overhead in a triumphant stance similar to DeNiro in *Raging Bull*.

Everyone erupted into wild applause for Lou, and especially so when Angela joined him in taking a bow. They stood together and accepted the homage. What a payoff!

Lou and Angela had come all the way from Las Vegas and brought the ingredients with them to lay out a complete dinner for twelve. As agreed, there it lay in all its splendor, with all the trimmings!

As I observed the happy couple basking in the much-deserved spotlight, my mind drifted back to the night in Las Vegas when I met them. I rarely stayed overnight in Las Vegas, but I had business there early Monday so I decided to spend the night at Caesar's.

After I settled in, I went downstairs for dinner. I stopped at the bar to see who was working. I knew several of the bartenders and waitresses as regular customers at the Crystal Cross. I had wanted to see them on their own turf, but didn't recognize any of the staff.

I ordered a drink and nursed it along, just killing time, when I noticed a commotion coming from a couple sitting next to me.

The bartender asked, "Can I get you anything else?"

The husband waved the bartender off with one hand while holding his head with the other.

The wife seemed a little self-conscious and embarrassed when she said, "No thanks, but thanks for the towel. You're very kind."

The bartender said, "No problem. Sure you don't need any help?" "No, really, we'll be fine."

I couldn't help but see how sick he was. I thought that perhaps

240

he'd had too much to drink. Then he turned and threw up again as he tried to get to his feet. This man wasn't drunk, he was obviously sick.

His wife said, "I'll get him to the room and it'll be okay."

The bartender brought another cold towel and set it in front of her husband. The man covered his face for a minute and then got to his feet, mumbling, "It'll be okay. Let's go, Angie. Thanks, pal. Thanks a lot," and then they left.

I had finished my dinner, stepped off the elevator, and turned the corner heading for my room when I almost bumped into a maid hurriedly coming out of a room with an armload of dirty towels. I glanced into the room and saw the couple from the bar.

The husband, now dressed in his robe, leaned against the wall as if bracing himself before he went into the bathroom. He couldn't make it before he vomited again. His wife supported him.

Over an hour had passed since I'd seen them downstairs. I stood no more than ten feet away when I said, "Excuse me ma'am, what's wrong? Does he have food poisoning?" I knew that I had my clay, and if it was food poisoning I had an answer.

"No, it's a migraine."

"A migraine? He's throwing up from a migraine?" I'd heard of how bad they could be, but at the time I'd never actually seen someone throw up because of a migraine headache.

"Have you called the house physician?"

"Yes, he came and gave him something, but it didn't help. He has a history of these migraines. It just takes time, usually up to six hours, sometimes longer."

"Six hours of this?" I hadn't yet talked to him but I knew that he could probably hear me. The maid came in with fresh towels. I asked, "Can he keep anything in his stomach?"

The man answered. "No, I can't."

"I'm sorry to disturb you, but I think that I can help. I know I can help!"

His hand came down from his head and he turned to me.

"Yeah? How's that, pal?"

I felt a bit awkward talking to a man so sick but I said, "Have you ever heard of Clay Therapy?"

He raised his head and asked, "What therapy?"

"Clay. Therapeutic Clay. I'm heavy into it."

He buried his face into the towel again and said, "No, don't know anything about it. Whattaya mean you're into it?"

"I have a Therapeutic Clay Center an hour and a half west of town. Clay Therapy is my business."

His wife said, "We never heard of such a thing."

"Well, it's all very real. I think it'll help. I've had some good results before with migraines. It's really common knowledge at my place."

He looked at her, then back at me. He didn't want to deal with me. I couldn't blame him.

"I carry it with me all the time. It's no problem. Nothing to it. I can get it in a second. Usually doesn't take but thirty to forty minutes to work, then that's it."

They looked at each other and jointly shrugged Italian style as if to say, "What's to lose?"

Then I added, "The price is right, too. I'll charge you a good bottle of Dago Red after it works."

His wife stepped forward to help him, as he was about to throw up again. As she did, he said, "You're really serious, aren't you pal?"

"Serious as your migraine."

He glanced up at me and asked, "What's the name?"

"Graham. Cano Graham from Tecopa Hot Springs, California."

He said, "Ca-ne?" He pronounced it Ca-knee. "What the Hell kind of name is that? Ca-ne means 'dog' in Italian." He was working the name bit pretty good. "Damn. A man named Dog with dirt for my head! And you got the stuff with you?"

I loved his act. "Sure do, Bud."

242

He countered, "And you say the fee is a bottle of Red? Well, I'll tell you this Dog, if you can stop this migraine in one hour, you've got yourself one thousand dollars. Payoff is tonight in crisp one hundred dollar bills. Ten of 'em, okay?"

He had a way about him. I certainly liked them both. I wondered what he did for a living.

I said, "First, it's Cano. Not Ca-ne, and second, about my fee, the payoff will be someday at my place, a home cooked meal to go along with the wine, for a dozen or so of my friends. Deal?"

His head was back in the towel when he said, "All your people can eat and drink." He leaned against the wall, so sick that he could hardly stand when he said, "What do I do?"

"I'll be right back. Get him into bed."

I quickly went to my room, three doors down, retrieved the clay, and returned to their room. I mixed up a glass of clay water, and put an ample amount of my clay on a wet washcloth.

"Okay, this is what you do. Sip some of this clay water, but go easy. Get as much down as you can. It's tasteless."

He was half serious when he said, "Dog, you want me to drink dirt? Jesus, man!"

"It's no big deal. People do it all the time. I don't have time to show you a medical book. Just do it!"

He shook his head in disbelief, but did as I asked him.

I put the clay-soaked washcloth over his forehead, eyes, and temples and beside his nose. I told him to leave it there for forty minutes. As I applied the cloth I gently pressed it into his forehead and into his eyes. "What's your name?"

"Lou. Lou Caruso from Chicago. This is my wife, Angie."

I thought he was about to throw up again. I said, "Relax Lou. Relax. Relax and try to nap for a few minutes. Shut everything off. We'll be right here."

Within thirty minutes, he had fallen sound asleep.

I said, "Mrs. Caruso, it's over. He's out of it."

She stood totally astonished. I was thrilled. He was resting easy. My self-esteem is never higher than at a moment like that.

"Mrs. Caruso, looks like dinner at my place. It'll be fun. Leave the cloth in place for an hour, cover him, and let him sleep. I'll see you in the morning."

The next morning as I ate breakfast, I heard a booming voice from across the room. "Hey! Dog!"

Angela tried to calm him down. He held his hands over his head clasped in a winner's salute. What a payoff!

I was thinking of that Sunday night and the next Monday morning, when he caught my eye and gave me a thumbs up sign, for the meal they'd produced.

He had his arm around Angela and smiled at everyone proudly. "Did we pull this off, or what?"

The dinner went wonderfully well. Lou steered a lot of new customers our way, and became a good friend. He'll get a kick out of reading his story.

Hi, Angie! Take care of my buddy.

Chapter 31

A Future Fish Fry

Imagination is more important than knowledge.   Albert Einstein

One Sunday afternoon, a month or so after Kuniko and the girls had been at the Cross, a sophisticated Japanese American businessman from Los Angeles named Honda approached me. He wanted to buy the Crystal Cross. At that time I had 20 acres and wasn't interested in discussing the matter. I certainly couldn't consider what I was creating to be put on the market and sold. Who would sell a child?

The next morning, before they left, he and his lovely wife, Noriko, let me know they had something of real importance to discuss, but preferred to explain these matters at their home in Garden Grove, California. I assured them I remained firm in my no sell position, but nonetheless they wanted me to have dinner and spend an evening with them.

They had a certain positive, refined, almost elegant quality about them, making it difficult to resist the invitation. Plus they lived about a half-hour from mother's home, and indeed he had succeeded in sparking my curiosity.

At their home the Hondas served a dinner of seafood like I've never experienced, and no one uttered a single word of business. When we finished they invited me to their den, which doubled as his office. After we settled into our chairs, he began the conversation in a most disarming fashion.

"Mr. Graham, you are not a businessperson, are you?"

I snickered, and shook my head slightly. Such a way to open what had to be some type of business meeting! He smiled as he waited for my response.

I chuckled and massaged my forehead while I formulated my thoughts. This had all the earmarks of the opening salvo of some kind of financial discussion, and he had just put me gently on the defense.

I smiled back at him. "Well, Honda san, that's some question, but then it's not really a question as much as a statement." I acknowledged his wife and said to both, "You're on the button. I'm in business, but I don't think of myself as a businessperson."

He leaned back in his chair, turned to his wife, and smiled. "Not many would answer that way." Still smiling, he shifted back to me. "Actually, we understood the situation the moment you refused to even consider my generous offer."

"Yes, it was generous. I'm simply not interested in selling."

"The Japanese have a saying that translated to English is much like, 'You have bigger fish to fry!'"

I laughed and said, "I thought Oklahoma had a lock on that phrase. But, yes sir, that is accurate. I do have an agenda."

"You want to build something don't you?"

"Yes, I do."

"As I thought! You're not a conventional businessperson, but more of a maverick developer, but even that doesn't really describe your motive."

He nodded to his wife and said, "She was the one who sensed your affection for the clay. It's all about the clay, right?"

I cracked a smile and scratched the back of my neck. "Certainly, the clay and what it will do is important to me, sure it is, and of course what I want to create."

"Since you won't entertain the idea of selling your place, and considering I have an interest in what your clay can do, I've decided to change tactics to help myself by helping you in a different direction. It has to do with marketing the clay."

"Honda San, I have no plans to aggressively market the clay at this time. I want to put all that business off until I have my place ready. Maybe in a year or so."

"Yes, yes, I understand. At the Crystal Cross you told me that Clay Therapy was your interest."

"I did?"

"Yes, you did. You said selling clay would come, but it wasn't important to you at the time." He included his wife when he said, "We only heard you mention Clay Therapy one time, but that was when my wife realized you weren't ever going to sell. We thought about it, and decided that if you had wanted to sell you would have shown us your projection of potential sales, but you didn't. So Mr. Graham, because of my interest, I have decided to take another road.

"The reason I invited you here was so I could introduce you to someone. This man has been my best friend since we were children in Osaka, Japan. Today he leads a large respected religious organization with branches all over the orient. He is the founder and owner of an extremely large pharmaceutical complex."

His smiles had fled, replaced with a quiet composed manner. He stood up and with a considerate gesture said, "Mr. Graham, please come with us."

With that said, he and Mrs. Honda led me into a small private altar. A softly lighted picture hung over the altar. It was his friend. I liked the feeling of reverence in their little sanctuary. We stayed for no longer that ten minutes or so while Mr. and Mrs. Honda prayed. After we returned to the den, Mr. Honda handed me a piece of literature that described his friend, what his business was about, and the extent of his religious organization. I was further intrigued when I realized they were a spin-off of Buddhism, since Buddhists weren't all that popular in Japan.

He referred to the literature when he said, "Mr. Graham, I've told him about meeting you, and of your particular clay, and he would like to know more."

"I'm impressed, and obviously honored to have such interest from a person like this. What would you have me do?"

"Mr. Graham, first I would like to have a written agreement that states if you export your clay to Japan, that my company will be the exporter."

"Honda san, I've never for a moment thought of exporting to Japan, or anywhere else, but if this materializes? Well, certainly, I would sign an agreement that you are the sole exporter to Japan of my clay. But he hasn't yet even used it to verify that the benefits I claim are valid."

"Very well, that brings us to the next point. He wants enough of your clay to thoroughly examine the results in several diverse applications. Naturally he will pay whatever is proper."

"Fine, no problem. All I need is his address, and I'll send him 50 pounds at no cost, with complete instructions along with a list of ideas he may want to pursue. I will have to think about the economics."

We concluded the evening with my head spinning. My base thought boiled down to the fact that it wasn't any shrewd moves on my part that brought this enormous potential to the surface, but rather the supreme integrity of this substance, pure and simple.

I spent the night at Mom's house and walked around the lake until late, considering the implications of the evening. Now I could see why he wanted me on his turf. He had me all along, but he didn't know it, or did he? .

With an attorney friend as my counsel, I began the communication with Mr. Makato Tanaka in Osaka, Japan. I did what I said I would do, when I said I would do it. Before too long he let me know that the clay had exceeded his expectations. I was elated with the prospect of covering the orient.

My attorney was less excited on the phone as he dryly

suggested, "Cano, why don't you come in, we need to talk about this Japanese thing. "

"Sure, no problem, be there Tuesday, if that fits."

"Fine, around 11:00, we can do lunch."

We talked about how things were going in Tecopa Hot Springs, what I intended to do up there, and he wondered when I planned to return to my acting career.

Out of the blue he asked, "Cano, can you account for all the money you're investing in your place?"

The unexpected question frightened and shocked me as though he had just splashed me with a bucket of ice water.

What was he asking me? Now the situation was fully out on the table.

"Account, uh, for my money? Like where it came from? Well, I've been meaning to talk to you about this thing. I've just been so busy that ..."

"Okay, settle down. I didn't think so. Look, Cano, what if the IRS starts to show an interest?"

"My, my, this sure is a cheery conversation."

"Cano, it's more dangerous than I think you know. I mean, if they ever start looking around or are made aware of your effort?" He played the devil's advocate, but at least I was beginning to get a clearer picture.

"For instance, in exporting the clay to Japan, have you thought about the strings that could come with such a decision?"

"Well I thought it could really put us on the map in one sense."

"On the map! That's the point. It probably would, and maybe get us a lot of press! Cano, you're an artist building a Clay Spa in the middle of nowhere, not far from Death Valley. Seems like a natural story, or natural iceberg. This could easily cause your boat to attract a lot of attention, but every inquiry could gouge a big hole in your vessel. Oh, my God man! You could take more rips than the Titanic if a problem ever started."

"Damn! I don't like that analogy."

Standing, he lit a cigarette. "Cano! You're already too visible up there. I mean, this could put you on the 6:00 news in Las Vegas. The IRS has snitches that look for new money. Do you have any detractors? I don't want to unduly scare you but I've been meaning to ask you about your tax situation. Are you…?"

I held up my hands and turned my head as if to protect myself from blows.

"I'm sorry, Cano."

"I know, I know, the Titanic." I was crushed.

The die was cast. I had to cease and desist with my Japanese friends. I was advised that I couldn't even afford the luxury of explanation. Just stop, back off completely, and hope it wasn't too late.

Mr. Tanaka in Osaka personally wrote me four letters, all praising my clay and wanting to do business. He must have thought me an unprincipled person.

I was knocked off balance. If I couldn't execute with the Japanese, then what next? How vulnerable was I? What about my future?

I pushed it all back and continued to build. I've since apologized to all my Japanese friends. I'm looking forward to a return engagement. Someday.

Chapter 32

Pearl

Man is certainly stark mad: he cannot make a flea, and yet he will be making Gods by the dozens. Michel DeMontaigne

One Sunday morning, I sat in my chair on the front porch with a Bailey's and coffee in my hand. I was just enjoying life and watching the customers.

Joyce came up behind me, put her hand on my shoulder and asked, "Cano, who are you expecting?"

I replied, "I'll know when I see 'em."

The action was hot and heavy. I loved it. I had just done a very successful radio show in Las Vegas, and we got in a whole new crop of people. Most of the people enjoying the Cross had come to relax, soothe an aching back, arthritic joints, or to satisfy their curiosity.

I had gotten into the mode of watching for those who had tried everything, but with no success. Word had gotten out about us and many people came to us who had grown tired of doctors, and drugs, and hospitals, and the health care system in general.

Later that afternoon, a late-model car drove up close to the office area and a well dressed a man and woman in their later thirties, got out. In the backseat sat a woman who looked to be in her mid 40s. Equally well dressed, she had dark brown hair with streaks of gray.

Someone had told her about us, or she had heard me on the radio. Either way, I sensed she had come to make contact with me, one-on-one. She had lovely, soft brown, intelligent eyes. She gave the impression of someone very serious, and I could see her focus on me. I didn't see her blink.

She had a problem, and I sensed she knew, almost like something preordained, that I realized we had something to resolve. Clearly, the activities and people were merely peripheral to our encounter. Only fifteen to twenty feet apart, we both sat still and studied each other.

The stuffy ones obviously belonged together. They radiated a stoic, aloof manner and one felt a cold, sterile, and uncaring core to them. Somehow they were tied to the one in the shadows of the back seat, and I felt it wasn't a humanitarian link

Goose bumps popped up on my arm.

The man and woman approached the porch, and the man asked, "You're Cano Graham?"

He made it sound like an accusation.

I immediately bristled. I didn't like these people. They knew more about me than I knew about them. I felt a bit defensive. I'm uneasy around people like these. They always take more than they give. They knew about me, my place, and what we did with the clay. I figured they also anticipated what to expect in return for whatever request was coming.

I reacted spontaneously by firing directly at his brain. "Yes, I am, and I'm so glad she decided to come." The forthright greeting indicated that I was fully aware of them being on the way to my place.

I knew this couple before I saw them, and the lady was like someone I had known 1,000 years ago. The couple glanced at each other, more of a twitch, really. I had leveled the playing field.

The woman, who could have been a model for a plastic mannequin, stepped forward, boss-like and asked, "What are your rates by the month?"

"Why don't you ask the woman in the back seat to get out so we can get acquainted? She's the one who wants to stay here. Isn't that correct?"

I sensed a definite electric barrier between us. I didn't particularly like either of them. I got up, walked past them to their car, bent over close to the window and said, "Hi! Glad you made it. Not feeling too good, huh?"

She showed no emotion as a tear slid into the corner of her mouth. The woman said nothing, and with her little finger, wiped the tear away. It seemed a noble surrender of some kind.

I opened the door, and offered her my hands. I could tell she suffered severe pain, but I couldn't tell where. She labored mightily just to get out of the car. With an almost superhuman effort she rose and grasped both my hands. I realized as I supported her, that she was trembling.

The first words were reflected in her beautiful eyes before she ever spoke. "Thank you. Thank you so much."

The mannequin pierced the moment with a cold, "How much are the rates?"

I said indifferently, "You don't want any literature, or to see our accommodations, or our services? You're only interested in the rates? I believe you already know how inexpensive the rates are. Why this inquisition? The important thing is that she's here! It's amazing to me that she got here. I don't know where ya'll are from, but I feel as if you've been on a cross-country journey to get here. We're talking about this woman's life, and your sole concern seems to be the rates, and you two aren't even paying the bill. Is that correct?"

Their silence validated my position.

I shifted my gaze back to this lovely person who bore up under tremendous pain. She waited patiently while I told her escorts exactly what I thought of them.

"So, it's up to you then. Are you low on funds?"

Her body language showed her discomfiture with the question

and the situation.

I turned to the woman who still held my hands. "First, ma'am, and pardon me for not asking sooner, by what name do you prefer to be called?"

She spoke in a voice that fit her eyes perfectly. She perked up a bit and said, "Pearl. I like to be called Pearl."

"Hi Pearl."

The two creeps just looked at each other as if Pearl had just made up her name.

I nodded and said, "Hmmm. That's a beautiful name. It fits you." In a capricious decision I said, "Okay, Pearl, you know there are no doctors here. This is a really rustic place, and right now we're building, but then, you can see that. I'm going to charge you twenty dollars a day. That will include the food I want you to eat, the hot baths, massage therapy, and the therapeutic clay baths. That's it, and naturally that includes your room. Let's not discuss the rates anymore. Okay?"

She was here and we were going to take care of her. Pearl was safe.

"There's only one condition that I'll ask of you, simply that you do what we ask, to get yourself well."

Barely perceptible, a smile broke through her pain.

"But I must ask now. What do you do? What happened? What caused all of this?"

She spoke for the first time. "I'm a commercial artist. I had a cancer operation six months ago. Since then, I've gained thirty pounds, and the doctors say that arthritis has infested every joint in my body. I can't work and it's getting worse."

I admired her poise. She had a courageous air about her.

"When do I start?" she asked.

"Pearl, I don't understand what I know about you, but I know this, the toughest chapter is over. You're here.

"Now then, this is the main routine: You get massages, hot mineral water baths, and gentle exercise twice a day. Then I want you to spread a sheet on your living room floor, make sure the heat is up, and cover your entire body with warm clay that's kept in a big crock in your room. Lie down and be quiet. No television. We have some great music for you to listen to if you like, but mainly I want you to focus on being well. Nothing far-out.

"Just quit thinking about the problem. The clay is going to attack the source of the problem, and it's going to draw the pain away. We don't yet know exactly how it works. Nobody does I suppose, but it does, and it will, no matter what you do. But it will be better for you to help it along. I want you to prepare for prosperity."

She remained calm, as if nothing I said surprised her.

"Pearl, I've got to go to Los Angeles and it may be a while before I get back. The staff knows just what to do, and I'll check on your progress often. Be sure to let the clay dry completely, twice a day, soak it off and then cover yourself with moisturizing cream."

Pearl's recovery bordered on the supernatural. After four days she was walking by herself. At the eighth day, she informed the staff that she was going to ask me if she could move there and become a permanent member of the staff. She really enjoyed working with guests who needed help. Outgoing, poised and cheerful, Pearl was a joy. She was fast losing weight and had become the talk of the community.

One afternoon, a staff member heard Pearl tell someone on the phone of her plans to move to Tecopa Hot Springs and join the staff of our Center.

"Don't you see? I can be of service and pain-free at the same time. I have a new life here! Please."

She was obviously interrupted in mid sentence. She instantly went out of character, became dejected and hung up the phone. That was the twelfth day of her stay. Someone would never know how badly he or she had hurt Pearl.

I returned two days later, fourteen days since her arrival. The first thing I noticed when I pulled into the parking area next to the office, close to her room, was the car she came in and the guy who had dropped her off.

When I got out of my truck, I saw Pearl carrying her suitcases to that car.

"Pearl?"

She stopped dead in her tracks, holding two big suitcases.

"Is that you?"

"Yes, Mr. Cano, it's me."

"This is incredible! Beyond anything I've ever seen."

She stood in a sheer, spring-like dress, with her hair pulled to one side. I was completely aghast. The creep took her suitcases. She was leaving?

I said, "Pearl, where are you going?"

The man glanced at me as he put her suitcases in the trunk.

She replied but stayed in motion, "I'm just going to town. I'll be back soon."

"Why are you saying that? You're not coming back. Not ever."

I knew what I knew. Not ever.

I was emotionally on fire. She looked so alive, so improved, so vibrant, but she needed more therapy. Her feeble excuse floored me.

"I'll be back soon."

I walked over to the car and approached her mannequin friend, who stood there looking sort of bored with all the dialogue. I said, "Pearl is doing so well!"

She looked as if she didn't appreciate the name Pearl to start with, and then in a casual, offhanded manner said, "Yes, she is better."

I wanted to slap her! "Better? Pearl has had a metamorphosis! Look at her! What's going on? Pearl, do you want to leave? Do you?" I felt dumbfounded, hurt, and confused. This was bad fiction at it's worst. What did they have on her that they could force her to

256

leave like this?

Pearl remained subdued.

I went ballistic!

She stiffened, and said in a pathetic manner, "I'll be back."

"No, you won't. You'll never be back. Not ever! Why are you doing this to yourself?" I looked at her two friends, and saw nothing in their expressions, their eyes, their mouths, nothing.

I asked a staff member to go and get a sack of powdered clay and I gave it to her. I said, "Pearl, this will last you a long time. Go easy. I'm sorry if it didn't work out for you, but you've made tremendous progress. You really look great! I'm proud of you and I'm happy for you."

I turned and walked toward the office, then wheeled around and went back. Pearl had already settled into the shadows of the back seat of the car. The woman sat in the driver's seat, and the man stood in the door ready to get in. I stopped, and suddenly something came over me.

"I'm curious. What religion are you folks?"

He said it like a robot, "We're Witnesses."

"Jehovah's Witnesses? Fine! Good to know that there are no doctors here, no chemicals, and no medical establishment, just healing Earth. So, why? Why?"

My rhetorical question hung in the air heavier than the Mercedes' hum.

Pearl and I locked gazes across that abyss and I felt connected to her by an invisible umbilical cord. Then she silently passed by me as the car slowly proceeded down the dusty road, and turned onto the main highway as if leading a phantom funeral procession.

I never saw Pearl again.

Chapter 33

The Charter Members

The artist appeals to that part of our being which is not dependent on wisdom; to that in us which is a gift and not an acquisition-and, therefore, more permanently enduring. He speaks to our capacity for delight and wonder, to the sense of mystery surrounding our lives; to the latent feeling of fellowship with all creation.

Joseph Conrad

The note came by certified mail and I anxiously signed for it. The exquisite invitation, a reservation for Mr. Cano Graham's party of four to attend a festive occasion, came with the compliments of the host at the Mirage Hotel and Casino. I noted the date of the event and read that I had to confirm with an R.S.V.P.

Well, now, party time at the Mirage? I had no idea what it was all about but figured I'd find out in due course. In the meantime, Hooya! I decided to take Joyce, Ruthie, and Mom.

I confirmed our reservations and on the appointed date, the four of us headed for Las Vegas.

Our unrestrained enthusiasm led us to initiate the party day well before we left Tecopa Hot Springs. As usual, Mom was the prime instigator, and served the girls wine around 3 p.m. I tried not to give any indication, but I had a few other troubling subjects on my mind, namely my biz was going through some severe hiccups.

I was antsy. Some of my people were nervous, and I had a constant eerie feeling that something was about to go wrong. I wasn't far off.

Anyway, I used this relaxing early November evening to enjoy a few quiet moments on my sanctuary called the Hill. We were definitely in the mood for having fun. For those of us who didn't dress up often, to do so was special and was genuinely a big kick. The girls, Mother again, decided our group would and should be as sharply dressed as any four in Las Vegas.

Joyce borrowed a lovely beige evening dress that mother had altered to fit her perfectly. The hue of the material seemed to be color coordinated to match her shoulder length, beautiful blonde hair. Mother caught us all by surprise though, by wearing a purple floor length outfit she had made. Ruthie was her usual fit-to-kill self, and was sporting a green and yellow pantsuit. Only Ruthie could wear this kind of thing. This female ensemble could stop traffic on the Strip, well slow them up anyway.

I wasn't doing too bad myself by bringing a more stable influence to this wild bunch of country girls. I was rather dapper I must admit, decked out in my ultra special navy blue blazer with charcoal gray slacks and matching tie, all in all, a conservative contribution to our radical foursome.

For the girls, I had ordered lovely corsages, plus a white carnation for my boutonniere. The flowers were delivered on time from Pahrump, Nevada and precipitated a certain excited crescendo among the girls.

We were ready and set to roll.

On the drive to town, we occupied ourselves by trying to figure what group was sponsoring the whole evening. We had long since worked ourselves into a fever pitch, when we passed in front of the Mirage. At that moment a huge eruption of fire and steam from the volcano blew right in front of us. I thought mom was going to bail out of the car.

"Hey, they didn't have to do that for us, ha! It's like a personal greeting. I'll have to remember to thank Steve for that."

"Who's Steve?" Mom asked.

"Steve Wynn. He's the owner of the Mirage," I replied.

When we entered the lobby, the maitre d' approached us and elegantly enquired, "Mr. Graham, party of four?"

I nodded and discreetly palmed him a twenty. He countered with, "Right this way, please."

This reminded me of a scene from a Cary Grant film.

The maitre d' led us into the main auditorium, which confused me. I didn't get it. We all looked at each other for some kind of support, but that was no help.

Then Mom said, "So far so good."

We all broke into peals of laughter. She sounded like a lady bank robber leading us in a heist of some kind. Then the pressure of the moment took a turn up, going from fun to frantic.

The previously noisy audience quieted as we found ourselves escorted through the crowd. All heads turned as we passed. It seemed as if the maitre d' was taking us on stage! We grew more self-conscious as each second passed, and I might add we loved every minute of it. Our adrenaline flowed like champagne. We all acted as if nothing was out of order, just another night out as the maitre d' led us all the way down front.

I still wondered, who in the Hell is putting this party on? I don't know anyone here.

But then Joyce said, "Cano, some of our guests from the Cross are here." She waved to someone, then to others.

I heard someone say, "There's Cano and his Mother."

Talk about excited!

Mother held tightly to my hand but looked cool.

I remember thinking, you can't let them see you sweat, but, man, this is fun!' Good Lord! This was like we had run a 21st Century gauntlet of some kind.

Coincidentally just as our party was seated, the orchestra's opening blast made us feel as if we were what they had been waiting for, which certainly wasn't the case.

Soon enough the audience realized that the opening music was simply a lead-in for the Master of Ceremonies.

The Master of Ceremonies came to the stage and announced, "A special anniversary request is being showcased by a prestigious member of the orchestra prior to the opening acts and the headliner. This request is not for a guest as such, but rather dedicated to the wife of the performer and some of their friends known as the 'Clay Disciples' from Las Vegas and Tecopa Hot Springs, California."

What had he said? "Clay Disciples?"

The emcee captured the audience's attention and piqued their interest with an unusual explanation of what we were about to experience.

"Our artist will perform Paganini's *Caprice Number 13 in B flat Major*, sometimes referred to as *Le Rire du Diable*, due to its mocking descending theme which some imaginative listeners interpreted as a devil's chuckle. Ladies and Gentlemen, since the artist has chosen a piece by the legendary Niccolo Paganini, it must be noted that Paganini intended this music primarily as a showcase for his phenomenal technique.

"The music you will experience is filled with the most dazzling and electrifying effects, in which technical complexity is glorified for its own sake without much regard for sound musical values. Paganini pieces represent charming melodic ideas and effective harmonies, but the interest this evening will be centered entirely on pyrotechnics. The digital feats called for by this music make the severest demands on the virtuosity of our performer."

I thought, in other words, if the artist didn't have the chops, then he or she couldn't handle this piece.

With this announcement a ripple of rustling apprehension wove through the audience, as they seemed to sense something truly special was about to happen.

In the most sophisticated and reserved manner the emcee

announced, "Ladies and Gentlemen, Mr. Abe Little!"

I thought, "Abe? Abraham?"

When he briskly walked toward center stage I recognized him instantly, tux and all! On the big stage he appeared shorter, but projected an accomplished, dignified and self-assured presence. He took his position as if he owned the space. The lights dimmed and a spotlight featured him on center stage. Joyce and I turned to each other with mouths agape in astonishment and mouthed, "That's Abraham?"

Mother pulled at my arm. "Honey, who is he? Is he a friend? I don't understand."

After a stunned moment I answered, "Yes Mom, he's a friend. You'll love him. He's been a guest several times at the Cross. That's Abraham! He has a wife named Muriel. They're the Littles, from here in Las Vegas. He's a Concert Master Violinist, but he's been unable to play. They thought that he was through, because of some syndrome, an injury from playing too much, too long, something like that. It's damaged his arm. My God, our clay healed him. He knew it would!"

I then learned that this day was Abe and Muriel's 40th anniversary, and that they wanted us to help celebrate the day and his recovery by having this party. As his performance started, a video of the day I first noticed them leaving the Crystal Cross began to play through my mind.

I stood talking with some friends when I noticed a particular couple appeared bursting with enthusiasm because of their mineral water and clay bath experience. I soon learned that this slight, balding, proper man was Abraham Little. His wife Muriel was a gentleman's lady.

I harbored an instant affinity for them, which was enhanced when I learned that he could do what I silently dreamed of doing. Abraham Little was a first chair violinist. I learned about his musical prowess when I inquired about them, and promised myself to get acquainted with them the next time they drove out from Las

Vegas. .

In our first formal introduction he said, "Mr. Graham, you'll never know just how much we value and appreciate these days we spend in the clay baths. We believe that through this place, with the water and clay, we'll be able to regain a way of life."

I thought, how much more serious can it get?

He had communicated something even beyond the words he was saying.

I said, "I believe I understand. You have some very personal reasons for feeling the way you do." I didn't know how to express what I sensed. "Oh, please excuse me, but would it be presumptuous of me to use the word *reverence* to describe your affection for our clay?"

His eyes moistened, and he laughed with embarrassed relief. He put his arm around me and gave me a reassuring and thoughtful hug and then his lovely wife Muriel did the same.

"What is it?" I asked. "What's at the very center? What's it all about?"

The three of us held hands as he thoughtfully and quietly explained. "I've been a musician, a violinist in Las Vegas for forty years and I thought it was over. At first my arm began to get sore and ache, a dull and sustained pain, but it often went away with a little rest. But now I can't get the pain to go away with the rest and it causes stress that affects every aspect of our life."

He glanced at Muriel and smiled briefly. "It's no longer a matter of my pain, but a matter of *our* pain." He rubbed at his right arm without thinking.

"I knew I wouldn't be able to work much longer, and it frightened me because it grew progressively worse. After a show or two I found that I was unable to go to sleep because it hurt continuously. The pain medication doesn't work and I've begun to experience severe depression, Mr. Graham. I had to put my violin down."

Muriel said in a whisper, "This is all such a blessing to us. We know that the clay and water will work."

I said, "I'll hear you play when you get through this. "

Abraham smiled and said, "I'd love to play for you and your friends, when I can. I suppose it will be in God's own good time." Soft, silent tears ran down his face.

The men I admire most are those with the capacity to cry. Then he laughed with the refreshing manner of someone who cries from joy. I'll never forget that magnificent moment with this artist and his lady. He laughed and brushed aside a tear. "Do you remember Heidi, the tall red headed girl who danced at Caesar's?"

I tried to remember. "Does she have a baby with red hair too?"

"Yes, that's her."

I had it. "She had bad feet. The dancing was killing her. Sure, I remember now. She was really a sight, she and the baby playing in the clay pools. I believe I had her cover both her feet with a thick layer of clay, put on socks and let them bake in the sun."

"That's right! That's how I found out about your clay. She saw me holding my arm, and asked me what the problem was. When I had explained the situation, she went into her apartment and brought out this big cookie jar filled with gelled clay, and began putting it on me right by the pool! Within a half-hour I knew that my prayers would be answered."

Muriel interjected, "Mr. Graham, you would just have to know how many doctors we saw with no results before you can understand this feeling we have."

Abraham continued, "Heidi gave me some clay in a bowl and suggested that I do it often, and told me about this place, and here we are. I recall that she referred to herself as a 'Clay Disciple.' Ha! She was some girl, and a terrific dancer. She moved to Reno. Did you know?"

"No. I didn't know that she had moved, but I'm so glad that she got relief. When the feet hurt, it all goes bad. It's funny how it works, isn't it? Someone told her, and she told you. The clay creates its own momentum."

Then he said, "Is this Clay Disciple thing a club or something? How do we get in?"

I hugged them both. "You're already a member, charter member."

I could still see the sparkle in their eyes when Mother brought me back to the moment by whispering in my ear, "I'm so happy and proud of you."

The sensation inspired me. To share this moment with Mother knowing that we were all seriously a part of the event dug deeply into our hearts. I smiled and acknowledged my three ladies, and they understood. Then I wondered if in some dimension our clay or the Power was aware of this moment. How could she not be?

What a moment. To know the despair he felt just a few months ago, and to now experience Abraham performing so beautifully that which he loved so much, and to share the moment with all his friends from Las Vegas, Los Angeles and those he had met in Tecopa Hot Springs!

Everyone in the room sensed that this enchanting experience was truly an inspired reflection of love and affection from this gentle man's heart. He played Paganini as few have. Abraham Little didn't play lovely music, he was love, and he was the music. The sounds and effects of that evening came not from his violin, but from God's instrument, and that instrument, Abraham himself.

One sensed that Paganini himself was just off the stage, unseen and smiling his approval. That night, Abraham was power plus. Waiters, bartenders, off-duty dealers, and floor men along with his audience exploded to their feet with deafening, appreciative and loving applause when he finished with a flourish.

Abraham held the hall spellbound. We had experienced a time to cherish always, an affirmation of life, a study of the Power in action.

Without so much as a deserved curtain call, Abraham then raised his hand and instrument to still the audience. Almost in the same motion he pointed his violin at our table and a spotlight singled out and covered Muriel. The audience knew and loved her, and did they ever show her how much!

After nearly a minute, the spotlight widened to include our group. Abraham motioned for us all to stand. Muriel rose to a thunderous response, and after a few seconds took my hand to join her, I wanted Mother to stand with me, but for a moment she was crying too hard, then she rose to applause. It was thrilling having Mom and Joyce and Ruthie on one side, and with Muriel on the other to raise our hands together. At that sight Abraham motioned for the rest of the audience to join us.

Simultaneously, the audience became something more than the sum total of its parts. We were giving to each other, and receiving-all we were, we gave.

Sheer joy, pride, and love for this demonstration of the Power filled the room. It was an inside job.

CB CB CB

At that time in 1990, none of us had ever heard of a malady called Repetitive Motion Syndrome. Now it's nearly an epidemic in the United States.

Chapter 34

The Last Dance

Reminiscences make one feel so deliciously aged and sad.

George Bernard Shaw

During the final few weeks leading up to Sylvia Burton's 84ᵗʰ birthday, the wheels of deception stirred enthusiastically in Tecopa Hot Springs. To achieve our ambitious, albeit hidden agenda, Ruthie and her *compadres* busily ferreted out information concerning the scattered, though admiring, flock of friends acquired over the years by our Sylvia. They relished executing this task under the unsuspecting nose of our victim.

A radical segment of our old timers fiendishly cross checked and coordinated data with Ruthie to locate old friends and invite them to Tecopa Hot Springs for a combined Reunion of Old Timers and Surprise Party for Sylvia's eighty-fourth birthday. On the target day, I drove to Sylvia's in the sparkling Chief to take her to dinner in Death Valley, as we had been planning for weeks.

When she came to the door, she said, "Hi, son!" Executing a nimble pirouette, she spun around with the poise of a ballerina and showed off her beautiful long red dress. I just knew she'd had that dress for years. As the lyrics in "Lady in Red" say, she was lovely and amazing.

Her twirling had a kaleidoscopic effect on me. I could see her from eighty-four to twenty-four. We enjoyed a slow drive to Death Valley and some good conversation over a fine dinner at the Death Valley Inn.

On our way back to Tecopa Hot Springs, I said casually, "Sylvia, how would you like to stop by the Schooner Room, and see who's around?"

She instantly responded, "Why I'd love it! Sure. I haven't been in there for a couple of years, since back when it was the Snake Pit. Long time ago."

When we pulled up to the bar it was obvious that something was going on. We could find no place to park close by, and so we had to walk a little distance.

Sylvia questioned so many cars. "I don't understand this. Must be a wedding or something. Would you look at all the cars! But who could be getting married? Seems I'd know."

As soon as we entered the room a raucous chorus blared out with a lively rendition of "Happy Birthday, Dear Sylvia"

Mission accomplished!

We'd pulled it off!

Ruthie and company had enticed a house full of Sylvia's old friends, many she hadn't seen in years, to make it an evening to remember one last time. These old friends from years past took their time relating memories about our Sylvia, and she told some stories about them too.

We were all in a festive mood when Sylvia took me by the hand and walked me over to a polished, quiet older gentleman. She said, "Cano, I'd like you to meet Allen."

When we shook hands I could see the family resemblances, and said, "Allen? Are you the Allen of Kitty Kitty-nice Kitty fame?"

Everyone within hearing range laughed when he retorted, "Yes, and you know what? I still don't like cats, especially in trees!" Then in a more subdued manner he said, "Sis has told me what you're doing with the clay. I've always wondered why

268

someone didn't do something with it. Cano, it's nice to meet my sis's second son."

"Thanks, Allen. It's a pleasure to meet you."

Mori, Art, and Luella kept busy with nametags and saw to it that everything ran smoothly. Mori had one last sting of his own for Sylvia. He and Ruthie had been announcing songs as they played Mori's collection of old 78-rpm records throughout the evening.

A large, rawboned, elderly man came quietly in the door, and Mori scurried to give him a special greeting. I could tell the man was apologizing for being late, but Mori assured him there was no problem.

The big fellow took off his Stetson and stood quietly, looking in our direction. Darned if his bearing didn't remind me of John Wayne. By the fuss in the crowd it appeared several knew him. The dance floor was between songs when Mori started an approving buzz through the guests by announcing an old favorite song.

The newcomer sauntered through the idle couples to our table, then bent over behind Sylvia and said, "Excuse me, ma'am, but that's a mighty pretty red dress. Would you care to dance with an old miner? They're about to play our song."

Sylvia hadn't seen this man in over forty years. For a moment she was confused and taken off guard, but just for a second or so. Then she held up both arms and screamed, "Red!"

"Hi, kid. Let's dance. Like I said, they're playing our song."

Like a schoolgirl, Sylvia fluttered out, "Oh Red." She turned to me saying, "Cano, this is Red!"

The big guy said, "Hi, Cano, could I leave my hat on your table?"

"No problem, Red."

By now the floor had cleared for these sweethearts and they danced to "Stardust." At first, kind of formal, until he looked down at her, smiled broadly, and said, "You're looking good, Kid."

269

With that she put her head on his chest and they moved effortlessly together, the way they had a long time ago.

છ છ છ

Nothing divine dies. All good is eternally reproductive.
Ralph Waldo Emerson

Chapter 35

The Wreck

Nothing can work me damage except myself; the harm that I sustain I carry about with me, and never am a real suffer but by my own fault.   St. Bernard

I lounged in my robe, almost ready to go have breakfast at the Miners Diner, and the weather looked gorgeous. Curt kept himself busy on the dozer moving some boulders, and as usual, I gently woke my beautiful crystals to play in the morning light. I decided to have a half-cup more of coffee, and catch up on the latest news about this guy Saddam Hussein who was trying to steal Kuwait. The phone rang and I grabbed the remote to turn the TV down.

"Hello, Crystal Cross."

"Yes, is Cano Graham there?"

"This is Cano, can I help you?"

"Mr. Graham, this is agent Lynch with the Drug Enforcement Agency in Minneapolis, Minnesota. Ah, Mr. Graham, I have a package with eighteen thousand four hundred dollars in front of me that's addressed to you."

My mind cut him off. In that microsecond, a huge silver guillotine, the leading edge of which was afire with sparklers of emotions came slicing down through my brain and divided my life into two halves. The first half consisted of my mother, friends, all I have been, all I had loved, all I was creating and all that could have been was in the past. The other half contained an alien, sticky mass that represented everything I couldn't see in the future.

I knew instantly this meant I was going to fall.

The crystals' reflections danced insanely through the paralyzing moment. In prison lingo, I'd just taken a big hit. I was in a bad wreck.

My life was tumbling downhill, and about to burst into flames. Off and on I'd imagined how a bust would happen, if ever. I thought of all kinds of ways, a fluke, a snitch, but never did I consider the event as a simple telephone call at seven a.m., and especially when I was having coffee and enjoying my crystals.

The sound in the room came back. I was in that space of time between the event and the denied reality. I stretched my neck muscles to the right then to the left and said, "Well thank you, if you'll just send me my money, there will be no problem."

"Yes, well, Mr. Graham, there is a problem in so far as we have reason to believe that this money is related to a drug conspiracy. Hello? Mr. Graham, are you there?"

I had laid my head back on the recliner and cradled the phone between my chin and shoulder as I watched my crystals.

I suddenly saw brighter colors and a quickness never present before, and I wondered why.

"Ah-ah-yes-yes I'm here, Mister…Mister…?"

He snapped out, "Lynch."

"Of course, Mr. Lynch. Is that spelled L-Y-N-C-H? Like a hanging?"

"Heh, Heh, yes, as a matter of fact it is."

I smiled to myself. "Interesting! You know Mr. Lynch, if this were a play, no screenwriter would ever give your character that sort of name. It just wouldn't work. I mean a name meaning 'hanging by the neck', a lynch mob! No, it conjures up something too evil. No writer worth his salt would give you a name like Lynch. Excuse me, are you there, Mr. Lynch?"

"I'm here. Mr. Graham, please put your interpretation of my

name aside. Is there anything you want to say regarding…"

"Excuse me for interrupting you Mr. Lynch, but considering the content of this conversation, and the fact that I've just acquired a new rhythm to my life, it behooves me to get about it. So, as much as I've enjoyed this information, the only statement I'd like to make is good-bye and good luck."

I hung up the phone, got out of the recliner, and restarted my crystals to dancing. Literally within thirty seconds the phone rang again.

"Hello, Crystal Cross."

"You're line has been busy."

It was Mom.

"Hi, Honey, yeah, someone wanting information. What's going on? Kind of early for you to call."

"Oh, it's nothing, but I was working in my flowers just a few minutes ago, when I suddenly remembered a dream last night. Honey, are you planning on driving much today?"

"No, don't plan on leaving town, just going to eat."

"Good, stay home!"

"Okay, Boss, but why?"

"Oh, it's silly, but I dreamed you had an accident in your truck. It turned over on you. It worried me."

"No problem here. But I'll be extra careful in my truck. Now don't worry."

"That makes me feel better. By the way, you won't believe how well my flowers are doing this year."

We talked. I watched the pixie colors flitting about the room, and let Mom tell me about her flowers.

Chapter 36

Busy Time

*When you put your hand to the plow, you can't put it down until
you get to the end of the row.*   Alice Paul

I had to confide in Curt what I was facing. He never broke stride.
Curt offered no commentary, no opinion, no advice, no nothing.

He only looked me straight in the eye and said, "Cano, I'm
sorry. How can I help you do whatever you intend to do?"

"Thanks, Curt. I don't know how much time I've got before
the other shoe drops. I've got Joyce helping mom, so she's in good
shape. Other than mom I've only got one thing on my mind, and
that's finishing the Cross so that the place is running when I go
down."

"It's that important to you?"

"I don't think I really realized just what this whole place and
Clay Therapy means to me until now."

"I kinda figured all along you felt that way. It showed."

"How about taking a break? Let's go to the Diner and have
breakfast."

Over breakfast at the Miners Diner Curt said, "Cano, I know
this is a real private time, but is there any chance it might be less
serious than you think?"

"Curt, I talked to the people out of state where the trouble

274

originated and, I'm sorry to say that all doubt was removed. I'm going down for sure and from where I stand it looks like a tidal wave coming at me."

"The fact is, we're a bunch of amateurs that found by trusting each other we could make a lot of money, and we did! Pay back is hell, and that's where I am."

As I recall that morning with Curt, I knew he wanted to have some idea of what was coming.

"Curt, I just don't know at this point what to expect, but I can't imagine more than a couple of years, maybe five tops."

He didn't raise his head. "I'm so sorry."

We ate breakfast and only discussed the job in front of us, preparing the Cross. I had heard some horror stories about the amount of time being handed out, but I didn't think it would apply to me. Still, in the back of my mind came the thought of running.

I bought a book about changing identities, but lined up against that fantasy was the reality that I'd never be able to see Mother again, nor could I ever go near my clay again, or do any theater anywhere. Besides, I might get probation or something like eighteen months. But regardless of what was coming, I couldn't and wouldn't live as a fugitive, not with Eva Graham alive and aware of the situation.

I knew that if we could finish the Crystal Cross soon, and have it operational, that no matter how much time I might have to serve, the Cross could function without me present. Curt and I knew exactly what was necessary. To get the permits for all the structures needed, we would have to first redesign and dig all new lines for water, power, and sewer system.

When we finished this, and the inspectors signed off and cleared us, we could then place our building online. At that point the Crystal Cross would be breathing in and out by herself, running as smoothly as her clay and on her own steam. All we needed was time. We got busy.

Chapter 37

The Suitor

With audacity one can undertake anything, but not do everything.

Napoleon

The news hit town like the first atomic blast. A Japanese group from Hawaii had just bought the Tecopa Hot Springs Resort, the nicest and largest of the four businesses in town. The resort had fourteen rooms, nice hot baths, over 100 R.V. spaces and 160 acres of land. Then the rumor swept through town that these same people wanted to buy 300 acres of commercial property in Tecopa Hot Springs as well as an additional 300 acres for a twenty million dollar Resort catering to the Japanese.

The news blew me away, but the closer I looked at the situation the more I realized that in the long run their interest might prove a tremendous advantage for the core of what I wanted to do. I knew I wouldn't sell the Cross or any of my property, but if they wanted to buy the Resort's 160 acres, The Delights Hot Spring's 40 acres, the 300 acres in Tecopa and build a 20 million dollar Destination Resort for the Japanese, well that could indeed be fantastic.

Two hundred acres in Tecopa Hot Springs would effectively surround my prime 100 acres, but before I finished a long walk, I was actually screaming with arms overhead and full of sheer joy. I realized that though I was going down, this bewildering circumstance would bring a world-class resort into town with the Cross at its center. I knew whatever they created would benefit our center.

I could make sure the Crystal Cross Therapeutic Clay Spa and Research Center would compliment their services. I held the prime high ground, yet far and away more significant was my supreme single asset of owning four of the seven major hot water wells in Tecopa Hot Springs.

However, one point about the purchase of the Resort by the Japanese didn't make sense, but I assumed they had taken this point into consideration. The county of Inyo had a moratorium on drilling any new wells, and I didn't know if the Japanese knew this or not. The result of this policy meant the owner of the Hot Mineral Water Wells, be that in quality, (gallons per hour), or quantity, (number of wells), possessed a commodity more important than land itself. In our area, you were only as good as your Hot Mineral Water.

I've never been a very good horse trader, I don't like to bargain. Still, because of one lurking issue, unless there was something I didn't know, I had them in a solid corner in one respect. If what I thought was true then they were checked before I ever met them.

I was aware from the time I got Curt started on the race of completing our present needs (before I fell), that the new water, power and sewer systems for our center would only suffice a few years at best before we'd have to expand them. I could only imagine the fundamental and massive expense the Japanese faced to satisfy the demands of engineering, and install all the infrastructure necessary, for their project. This being the case, I had clear reason to believe the Cross could benefit in several critical areas from their sophisticated effort.

Though almost out of time, and running on a wing and a prayer, I knew that even though they owned the bank, I figured I had control of the vault, the water, and prime land.

The dance begins.

The realtor from Pahrump, a nice hard working guy representing the Japanese interests, called me. "Hi, Mr. Graham, this is Ray Turner in Pahrump. How ya doing?"

"Hey, Ray. Good! I hear you've been busy over here. Man, you're causing quite a stir."

"Well as you know, or maybe you don't, he's from Honolulu. Hawaii. His name is Akire Sato and he represents people with big bucks, and some exciting plans. It looks like a real windfall for the area, and could be a real bonanza for you."

"Wonderful! We need a break, and it sounds like he's the man. You know Ray, for him to snatch up the choice resort property first off proves he's serious enough."

"He really is, but the best part for everyone is that he's really being generous with his offers. No questions about that!"

"Ray, that's so good to hear, I wonder how or why he ever got interested in Tecopa Hot Springs?" Now I glanced outside, and saw Curt talking to some happy clients that normally wouldn't be in town this time of year if it weren't for the Crystal Cross.

"Ah-a, Mr. Graham, I don't really know just how he got interested. He didn't say. He just feels they can make something work if they pour in enough capital."

I thought, yeah right! I'm sure you have no idea. The Crystal Cross is making it happen now and we all know it! Somehow they heard about us, and that's why he's here.

"Anyway Cano, he's going to be in town again in three weeks and wants to meet you and make an offer for your property."

"I haven't thought much about selling, but who knows? I'd sure like to meet him, and maybe we can come up with something."

"Fine. Let's see, this is the third and he'll be here on the 21st. How about I bring him over and you two can talk?"

"Sounds good, and thanks, Ray."

The Proposal

With the purchase of the largest place in town, the instant effect on our little community reminded me of a fierce hurricane plowing through a thatched hut village. The rumors flew from the hot baths to the bar to the Miners Diner, to the Post Office, and back to the Hot Springs, and those rumors were diverse.

He was going to buy and close Tecopa. Where would the people who lived in the little apartments go?

He was building a gated resort, designed for the Japanese tourist and hiring all Japanese help.

These rumors created a problem because they all seemed plausible, because we all knew Las Vegas has a large Japanese tourist trade, as does Death Valley. Art, Sylvia, and Ruthie sat in my front room, very seriously concerned about the prospect of being uprooted. I assured them that if push came to shove they could all move onto my property because I wasn't selling, no matter what! They wanted to hear me say it, and I did.

They pulled in right on time. Ray Turner introduced Mr. Sato. The three of us enjoyed some small talk, and I served some coffee. Ray soon disappeared to walk around the grounds and left us alone. Mr. Sato was a heavy set, confident, and jovial person. Younger than me, I figured he'd be tough in a street fight. When I sat with him one on one I sensed a strange attraction, a kind of love-hate relationship.

Indefinable at best, I thought I felt the way a man would feel being introduced to his wife's lover. I could identify with his feeling about the place, but how dare this man enter my domain! Would they like him better than me? How could he be here, and me gone? He didn't love this place; he only wanted the real estate. This place loves me, and only under duress would the area allow him to have his way. He'd toss it all away for a price. "Mr. Graham, I've been told you like to get right to the point. That

279

being the case, I would like to discuss the possibility of buying your one hundred acres."

I pointed outside. "Sato san, as you can see we're in the middle of a building program, and frankly I'd like to finish my plans."

"What exactly are you building?"

"A Global Clay Research and Healing Center."

"A Clay Center?" He passed over the subject and asked straight out, "Mr. Graham, are you prepared to entertain a serious offer?"

Something in the way he said it offended me, and I wondered just how tough he was. I lost that thought and said, "I'm prepared to listen."

"Very well, I don't want to drag this thing out by offer and counter offer. I'd like to make you one solid offer to prove conclusively that I'm serious, so I can move on to other things."

"Sato san, I'm glad you feel that way. Just what do you have in mind?"

"Mr. Graham, I'm prepared today to put a signed offer on the table of $500 thousand for your 100 acres."

I had paid about $250,000 for my land, and invested $60,000. I had to pay the balance off in 10 years, but then he knew all that. He knew that his offer meant to net me a quarter million dollars. Whew! The offer beat shooting pool if you don't shoot too good! I said, "That would be cash?"

He nodded. "Cash." Then he stood. "Mr. Graham, I'm returning to Honolulu in three days. I'm at the Dunes."

"Sato san, I appreciate how you've approached this matter and out of respect for your time, and mine, I should let you know now, before you go to any trouble that I'm declining your very generous offer. Sir, I want to finish what I've started." He never even changed his expression. "I was afraid of that." Then he smiled. "I had heard you were very involved here. Well, Mr. Graham, thank you for your time."

After the dynamic duo left, I thought, what the hell did I just do? I'm going down. I could take the money and run! Damn, I'm in a Wewoka switch! Whew! It's time for some *vino*, or something!

At three o'clock that afternoon Ray Turner called back. "Mr. Graham, are you aware that Mr. Sato is waiting to negotiate. He thought a counter offer was coming."

"Nope. He said no messing around so I didn't. That was it, done deal."

Ray said, "Cano, that was just the first offer."

"Look, Ray, what's the point? He did what he does, and I did what I do. He offered, and I refused. Ray, I just want to build my place."

Ray said, "Cano he knows that! And he wants to meet again at the Dunes."

"He knows I'm serious about my place? And he wants to meet again? When?"

"Tomorrow at noon."

"Tell him I'll be there, and on time."

At 11:45 AM I walked into the Dunes and called his room. His lovely wife joined us for lunch and he quickly opened with a frontal attack. "Mr. Graham what do you want?"

"I want to build my Therapeutic Clay Center, but please understand Satosan, I would genuinely like to have you here. Your development could mean everything to this community. Sir, you tell me if I'm wrong. I believe you're completely informed as to what I'm about, and what we've created at the Crystal Cross. I also believe you realize my operation redesigned and upgraded, could be an important part, if not the pivotal issue in bringing your project together."

"Go ahead, Mr. Graham."

"Sir, let me be candid with you and your wife. You could duplicate my efforts easily enough in terms of the clay spa. You don't actually need my central twenty acres or my other 80 acres to complete your project. You bought or at least are buying the biggest, most modern place here. I don't know how much hard cash you've put down, but I do know the Resort and the owner. The place you bought has everything but the one thing it needs most."

"And what is that Mr. Graham?"

"I'm sorry, but what you need more than land is a good Hot Mineral Water Well. You may not have completely known about the situation when you made the deal, but I figure you do now. Sir, you don't have enough hot water to adequately meet your present needs, much less expand or build." He looked at his wife. They knew I knew. "Satosan, I'm serious when I say, I want you here! Let me help your effort, so that I can achieve my goals."

He turned to Mrs. Sato, smiled fatalistically, and said, "I believe he has a plan."

"Okay, here it is in broad strokes."

"In the what?" The idiom confused him.

"Sorry, the general idea. Anyway, I hold onto my twenty acres, and you underwrite or loan me on a twenty year note all that's necessary to complete my project, but all within your master plan." I slowed up to see if he was with me.

"Go ahead, Mr. Graham."

"In return for this consideration, I'll agree for you to have access to all the hot mineral water necessary for your project in perpetuity, and sell you the eighty acres for one dollar."

I saw no emotion in his face when he looked at Mrs. Sato then back at me. "Interesting. You're suggesting that everything in the Clay Spa would be designed into, and actually be a part of our services, but owned and managed by you. All engineering, architecture, all infrastructure, building, everything? We get the needed water for our purpose and eighty acres?"

"Satosan don't forget you didn't stop me when I suggested that the success of my Clay Spa precipitated your interest in the area, and that same success would also be the draw for the rest.

You have all the other profit centers. I have the Clay Center, and it's just a loan, secured by the Clay Center."

"Mr. Graham, it has been a pleasure for Mrs. Sato and myself. I'll take this offer back to Hawaii and see how my people feel about it."

"Thanks. I'd appreciate as quick a reply as possible." We shook hands, bowed a bit and said, "Sayonara."

They offered me $750,000 cash for all one hundred acres, and they would build the Clay Center as agreed. In addition, they would give me a 20-year contract to manage the Clay Center with an attractive salary.

03   03   03

I didn't lose. I ran out of time. Seventeen days later the U.S. Government seized my 100 acres. With this news, Mr. Sato backed off the resort and was never seen again.

Chapter 38

Working on Shares

No matter how old a mother is, she watches her middle-aged children for signs of improvement.   Florida Scott Maxwell

I spent the weekend with mom. Being with her and away from everything helped me relax. The government had seized the Crystal Cross. In my sleep, driving, watching TV, walking, no matter what or where, I knew my days with mother were numbered. She was so happy. It tore my brains apart to think of her alone without me to care for her.

I was losing ground emotionally and physically. I often had the same frightening nightmare, of being in some kind of quicksand, and mother crying. I found it difficult to rest. I stayed up late, and didn't take care of myself. Some nights I walked until almost daylight thinking about the answers that weren't coming, and always about the inevitable day when I'd go under.

Each morning I woke with a start, followed by a surge of cold fear that caused my pulse to race. I began to shy away from the days. The news from out of state couldn't be worse. Everything was collapsing.

The fracture started with a fluke, but this one misstep, four levels down from me, was causing the entire foundation to crumble. This was no explosion, but a classic implosion. We were caving in. The Government busily put their case together, and I had little time left, though I didn't know how much.

One day I sat in my robe watching *CBS Sunday Morning* with Charles Kuralt while Mother did some laundry. I smiled when I heard her let out a big "Whoopee!" She was feeling extra special since we were going to one of her favorite spots for lunch, that being Mt. Baldy Lodge in the San Gabriel Mountains.

She came down the hallway waving her discovery and saying, "I found two more in the wash! Honey, you need a billfold, something to keep your bills in besides a money clip. It seems like almost every time I wash your things I find 'em." She walked over to me and said, "Would you look at this? This is six I've found in the last month. You're going to have to be more careful! Five-dollar bills don't grow on trees you know."

Ever since starting my little side Biz I'd been collecting five-dollar bills. Whenever I broke a twenty or whatever, I crunched up every five-dollar bill and put it in my back pocket. Every time, and this went on for almost five years. At night I'd take the crumpled bills out and shove them in a sock. This was my money. Not for supplies, not for food or personal needs, not for Biz. I called it my retirement fund, and I just kept on socking the fives away. It would amaze most people to know how many five-dollar bills all crunched up, a big sock would hold. Furthermore, a stretch sock will swell up like you wouldn't believe. Awesome sight.

When she handed me the two fives, it reminded me of what I'd decided to do. My greedy attorney *friend* wanted more money. He had made me believe he could save me. That's a whole other sick story. I'll meet him again someday. Anyway, I didn't want to touch my main funds so I decided to use my fives to meet the attorney's ten thousand-dollar demand. By this time I had several big long socks packed solid in my storage locker. I had to determine how much I had in those socks, and the easiest way to estimate real close would be to weigh them.

I knew that each bill weighed approximately one gram, so it

would be a simple matter of doing some math, 28 grams per ounce, 16 ounces per pound, etc, so I weighed about $10,000 worth of my fives and realized I didn't want to unfold and count $10,000 worth of five dollar bills!

On the way to Mt. Baldy I said, "Honey, do you remember when I went to pick blackberries in Maud with you on shares?" Maud, Oklahoma billed itself as the Blackberry Capital of the world, and that distinction always impressed me.

She laughed and said, "Do I? I guess I do! You were so excited about helping me. You liked the idea that when we picked two boxes the farmer got one, and we got to keep one. You understood what 'on shares' meant real quick. Oh, honey that's a memory. As soon as you filled two little net baskets, you'd go to the farmer's table, push one to him, and say, 'One for you' then you'd tap your chest and say, 'And one for me!'"

"I remember. How old was I then?"

"Oh, about six or seven. You were a good little worker. You ran around and scurried under the bushes where the adults couldn't go. You were so afraid the other people would pick 'em all before we got what we wanted."

Then she laid her head back on the seat, and really started laughing. She got me laughing just watching her and I said, "I know what you're laughing about."

She shook her head, and still laughing said, "No you don't."

"Yes I do! You're laughing about when I got stuck under the darn blackberry bush. The stickers had me so I couldn't move either way."

"Yes I know, everyone was trying to get you free, but you wouldn't move. You just kept saying 'Momma! Momma! Ouch! Ouch!'" Mother wiped her eyes. "Oh my, we had quite a day. What made you think of that? I mean of us picking berries on shares?"

"Well, I need some help. This man owes me a lot of money and he's ready to pay, but the problem is, its' all in five dollar bills, and they're all wadded up."

"All wadded up? Why?"

"I don't know, they just are."

"So? What's wrong with that?"

"Well I just don't want to sit around, unfold a big bunch of five dollar bills, and then count 'em. You could sort of work like on shares."

"On shares?"

"Yes. Look, honey, if you'll help me, here's what I'll do. Every time you count out a hundred dollars then you get to keep five dollars. "

She loved the idea. "How much is there to count?"

"Oh, I imagine you could make a couple of hundred or so, maybe more."

"A couple of hundred! My Lord yes! When do we do it?"

"How about this evening?"

"Fine. Wonderful! Ha! Imagine that, counting five-dollar bills on shares. My goodness, whoever heard of such a thing?"

That evening while mom took her bath, I unpacked approximately ten thousand dollars worth of five-dollar bills on the kitchen table and fluffed them all up. She was beautiful in her special purple housecoat, and excited about the task. I knew she would've enjoyed the evening just as much, shares or no shares, because we were together.

Somehow she didn't consider what a pile of ten thousand in fives, (all crunched up), would be like, but then who would?

Mom said, "Okay, honey I'm ready. When do we start?"

"How about right now?"

"Now? Where are they?"

"On the table, you're standing next to 'em."

She turned her head, saw the huge pile of five-dollar bills all wadded up, and almost actually fainted. Using both hands she grasped her head and chest at the same time saying, "Oh, my Lord, I never saw such a pile of money." She had to sit down to catch her breath.

"Do you think we could have just a little glass of wine? Oh goodness, I hope nobody robs us!"

I kissed her cheek. "I think we're safe and I also think a glass of wine would be in order." I went to the fridge and was pouring the glasses when I said, "If you'll let me do just one thing? I need to get on the phone for awhile, do you mind counting by yourself?"

She laughed and said, "Oh no, Mr. Graham. I don't mind at all! Ha, just the opposite! I'm like you were picking berries! I was afraid you'd count faster than me! You mean I can count 'em all?"

On my last day on earth I'll remember mom, counting '85-90-95-100!' Then she softly patted her $100.00 stack, took a sip of wine, tapped herself on the chest as she picked up a $5 bill and said, "And one for *me*!"

Chapter 39

The Dunsmuir Spill

We never do anything well till we cease to think about the manner of doing it.
                                                        William Hazlitt

On a warm night in the mountains of Northern California, in July 1991, a Southern Pacific Railroad tank car jumped the track and fell directly into the headwaters of the Sacramento River. At 11:00 p.m., 20,000 gallons of the herbicide metam sodium flowed from the ruptured tank car into the pristine, trout-filled river. Three miles downstream is the railroad town of Dunsmuir, California. Their community is noted for three things: the Railroad Center, trout fishing, and fine people.

These mountain people slept with their windows open wide that night, unaware of the silent cloud of toxic gas that hovered above them and drifted through their homes. .

Early the next morning, they woke to something obviously very wrong, a chemical disaster. Hardy, active people woke with swollen, burning eyes, terrible headaches, and stinging ugly sores started to appear. The doctors were helpless to treat them, for they knew of no satisfactory antidote for this type of chemical poisoning.

The police blared warnings for the citizens to close their windows, and stay indoors. Meanwhile the Highway Patrol told travelers on State Highway 5 to roll up their windows and keep driving.

They said, "Don't stop in Dunsmuir."

It turned out that everything was killed for forty-five miles downstream from the point of contamination. The nightmare was real. There had indeed been a chemical disaster.

When the Dunsmuir Spill happened, I found myself very busy and running out of time—legally. Although I wanted to prove to myself and to the medical community what the clay would do against pesticide and herbicide poisoning, I knew it would take more of my time than I could afford. So, I just kept reading about the pain and destruction of the infamous Dunsmuir Spill. Frankly, I thought surely in time it would just fade away. I imagined the terrible symptoms would diminish, and everything would go back to normal, but that didn't happen.

The *Los Angeles Times* reported children had ugly sores on their bodies; women experienced multiple periods; and steady grinding headaches were driving people to despair. Many suffered from persistent rashes and bleeding gums. Malaise and fatigue were a daily part of what before had been active lives. Some had much worse symptoms than others. Miscarriages increased, and mothers were concerned about the futures of the unborn. A behavioral syndrome involving bad attitudes among family and friends caused squabbles and fights where there had been none before. Constantly aching muscles, painful joints, and sleepless nights had become commonplace for these hardy people. Worse than anything for these proud, fiercely independent people was the fear. Dunsmuir was a frightened community.

The medical establishment suffered from a reactive wait and see attitude. No one could really blame them, because they just didn't know what to do. Three months later, the people of Dunsmuir still suffered myriad symptoms.

Then, in September 1991, I read an article in the *Los Angeles Times* that described some very unattractive reactions to the

Dunsmuir Spill. First, the Southern Pacific Railroad ignored their culpability in the disaster, and stonewalled the media. Second, the City Fathers displayed an appalling insensitivity in downplaying the entire incident. They apparently didn't want to scare away tourists, or the dollars they bring with them. In addition, they tried to make injured residents look like low-lifes for applying for compensation. The whole scenario smelled noxious, like festering greed.

These revelations caused me to pack my truck with a large quantity of my clay and begin an odyssey which lasted, on and off, for a month. I soon learned a great deal about clay therapy and chemical poisoning.

Nick and Boyd (Two Brothers And The Lady)

When I got there, it looked peaceful enough, but as soon as I checked into a motel, the story started to unravel. A young man about sixteen years old sat behind the motel desk, reading. I saw a TV station truck from the CBS affiliate in San Francisco parked just outside.

I had read about the sores on people, and the constant headaches, but by this time I seriously wondered if these problems had lessened along with all the other symptoms that had been reported. Wrong. The first thing I noticed as I set my bag down in the lobby, were the sores on the young desk attendant's face. He looked as though he had grown used to them.

He asked, "May I help you?"

I tried hard not to stare, and wondered if I'd be able to help him. "Yes please, I need a room for a couple of weeks."

"Sure. We've got lots of rooms nowadays."

I understood.

"Are you a lawyer?"

I coughed slightly. "No, I'm no lawyer. I agree with Mr. Shakespeare."

He didn't get it. "What? Are you a newspaper man?"

"No, I'm not a writer, either."

"Huh? What are you then? I mean, excuse me sir, but why are you here? We're standing 200 feet from the river right now, and that spooks a lot of people, so I'm just sort of curious about why you're here. I mean, very few people come this way lately."

"To be candid with you, I'm here because I think I can help those sores."

"You're a doctor?"

"I'm no doctor, either."

He acted like our conversation had become a guessing game. He raised his hand as though in a classroom, "I got it. You're a-studying us, like those folks from the University?"

"Nope, I'm none of those things, but I do believe I can get rid of those sores on your face."

"Really?"

"How long have you had 'em?"

"From the start of the whole thing."

"What've the local doctors done for 'em?"

"Nothing they can do. You don't know nothing about what's going on, do you? Where'd you come from? Are you sure you're not a lawyer?"

"Nope! I'm damn sure no lawyer! Why do you keep asking me if I'm a lawyer? On second thought, I'm tired and sleepy. I want to crash. We've got a long way to go, and everything can't be done in a night."

"Yes it can! Everything can be done, or at least undone in one night! It's like we went to bed in one world, and woke up in another!"

His remark startled me. I paused a second, thought about it, and decided to sleep. "See you in the morning, son."

He asked in a rather hopeful tone, "Do you really think you can take the sores, rashes and stuff away? Now, just how are you gonna do it?"

Maybe because I heard the hope in his voice, I don't know,

but whatever it was I couldn't let it go. For almost four years I'd seen my clay heal gross infections, exotic rashes, and strange sores that nothing known to conventional medicine could touch, so, it was time to get busy. I couldn't sleep anyway, not with his skeptical refrain, "How are you gonna do that?" ringing in my head.

I started for the door. "I'll be right back."

"Where you goin', Mister?"

"Just going to my truck for some stuff." When I returned, I had a big cookie jar of gelled clay, and a big bag of dry, powdered clay. "Does it itch?"

"Itch? Mister, this stuff drives us all nuts! For some, it's worse than for others, but yes!"

"When are you off duty?"

"I'm off right now. The night man is coming on. My parents own the place, and we live here. Anyway, it's 7:45, and he comes on at 8:00, so I'm free."

"Have you got any plans?"

"Is that the stuff that helps? Ah, no. Excuse me. Mister, I mean my plan is to do whatever you ask me to."

I swear he had a kind of Huck Finn look about him and I liked him.

"Great, okay now, some of this stuff is a dry powder, and some is gelled. See?"

"Yes, sir. What do I do?"

He was anxious, and I was tired. "Put about a cup of this powder in a hot bath, and just soak in it. By the way, do you have a headache right now?"

"I've always got a headache. A lot of people do. My mom is real bad!"

"Are your parents here right now? If they are, go get 'em for me."

"No, sorry, they went to Redding and won't be back 'til tomorrow afternoon."

293

"Well, in any case, here's what I want you to do. First, get me a glass of water and a wooden spoon."

"Okay, I'll be right back!"

I had him put about a tablespoonful of the powder in a glass of water. "Mix it up." He did, then I said, "Drink it all down."

He looked at it and sort of hesitated. "What's in this stuff?"

"Trace minerals. Good stuff."

In a cavalier fashion, he tossed his head back, and there it went.

I looked at that glass. "There's some left in the bottom. Get some more tap water and swish it around. Get it all in your system."

He did, and smacked his lips, "Nothing to it. Doesn't taste like anything. It's nothing."

"Okay, now here's what I want you to do. Run a nice hot bath with a cup full of the clay."

Then he questioned, "Clay? Clay? Clay? C-L-A-Y?"

"Yep. Also, when you take your clay bath, I want you to put some of the clay on a hot, wet washcloth, get it all wet, and put it on your face, press it on your forehead, and over your eyes. Just leave enough space to breathe! Stay in the bath for forty minutes to an hour. Got it?"

"Sure, no problem." He stuck out his arm, and rolled up his sleeve, "Do you really think it will do something for my headaches, and this rash?"

"We'll see."

"Did you know that a lot of us who live near the river have got this darn rash all over our bodies?"

"I've read about that."

He went on, "I mean *all* over, and it's miserable."

"I'm sure it is. There's also something else I want you to do."

"What's that?"

"Are you going to be up for a while tonight? Say, 'til ten or eleven?"

"Sure, my little brother and I will be watching TV tonight. There's no school tomorrow. By the way, my little brother doesn't have headaches, but he's got the rash all over him, real bad. How about if I give…"

"No problem. Give him the works. How old is he?"

"Nine years old, and the itching really bothers him, and it stings too."

"For sure, but I've changed my plan a little bit. Here's what I want you to do first. I want you to put this gelled clay all over the rash and sore spots. Is it on your back?"

He whipped off his shirt. His back was covered with a painful looking rash.

"My little brother is the same, or worse, because he scratches them at night. Will it stop the itching?'

"It should, but let's get this straight first. Put it on every place that needs it, and on your brother's back. He can put it on yours for you. Just spread it on like a salve. You don't have to rub it in. Just cover the bad spots, okay?"

"Got it."

"Fine. Now then, let it all dry. You also might want to lie on sheets so it doesn't get on your mom's chairs, or the sofa. It'll wash right out, and won't stain anything, but there's no reason to be messy. Do you itch all over?"

"Mister, my brother and I have got this rash in places we've never seen before!"

I laughed. The youngster had a way. By now, I was really getting tired.

Then his youth came to the front again, "This is going to be fun. How many times do we have to put it on before the itching stops, and the headaches go away?"

The faith of children is inspiring. Adults always have all sorts of questions.

"It may take some time, but, right now you've got plenty of the powdered and gelled clay, and if I don't get to bed soon…"

He was pumped up, "You really believe this clay stuff will help?" He smiled ear to ear in response.

"Yes, son, I do believe it will help."

He wanted to hear it again. I liked him, and wished his folks could be there. I was sure they'd be very proud of the way he was handling himself.

"Do you want my brother to drink some, too?"

"I sure do. The works." I stood on the verge of exhaustion. "First cover yourselves with the gelled clay and let it dry. Then take a long bath with clay in the water, and use a clay-soaked washcloth on your face."

"Can I put the clay cloth on while I'm drying the stuff? You know, rather than waiting to do it when we soak?"

"Sure, go for it. Put it on the problem areas first, and then let it dry. You might want to turn the heater up a bit so you'll stay warm. When you soak in the bath it will take most of the clay off, but it will leave a slight film on your body. Let it stay, it will feel real good, and smooth. If some of the clay sort of sticks to the sores, it's okay, just let it stay on. The 'lady' just doesn't like to turn loose of a problem."

He smiled at the term 'lady.' "Yeah, right."

"You just might see a difference by tomorrow morning."

"Really?"

"Could be, but son, by the way, what's your name?"

"Nick, and my little brother's name is Boyd."

We shook hands. I sure liked him. "Anyway Nick, I've got to get some sleep, okay?"

"You didn't tell me your name, Mister."

"Oh, sorry. Cano. Cano Graham. You and your little brother have fun, and I'll see you tomorrow, Nick."

"Goodnight, Mister Graham."

We were friends.

I took a quick shower, and fell into bed knowing it had been a long, but fruitful day. Fourteen hours of steady driving, but what a great way to end my first night in Dunsmuir. I already had my lady working, and as always, it felt good!

Nick and Boyd were probably laughing, and smearing the clay all over each other by now. I always have the sensation of introducing a close friend to someone when I turn them on to clay.

I slipped into a deep sleep and awoke to the phone ringing. Where am I? The phone just kept on ringing. With closed eyes, I fumbled for the receiver.

Like a zombie I mumbled, "Hello?"

The excited voice on the other end assaulted my senses. I didn't want to deal with an excited voice. I wished it would go away. Why were they calling me? Who was it?

"What's gone?"

Now the voice yelled at me. "*It's gone!*"

I thought my truck had been stolen. "What's gone? Dammit anyway. What time is it? Who is this?"

"Mister Graham, sir, this is Nick. Downstairs. It's gone, sir! It's only been an hour. We didn't start putting the stuff on until 9:30, and it's 10:45 now, and *it's gone! My headache's really gone*! I've already called a couple of my friends. They've got the same symptoms and they can't believe it. They want to know what's in this lady. Ha! Can they get some?"

By now I sat up on the edge of the bed, fully awake. I rubbed my eyes, and laughed at the scene that played out in my head. He had called her 'the lady' again.

"Hey Nick, does this lady go to work on this stuff, or what? Three hours in Dunsmuir, and she already has a big win."

"Sir, you talk like she's really alive!"

"Could be, son. Could be."

"I know I'm gonna stay with the lady 'til her wheels fall off," and then he started laughing at his own joke.

I asked, "What are you doing now? Have you soaked?"

Still laughing he said, "We're both soaking. We're both soaking in the tub, with the phone. Mom wouldn't allow this if she were here, but, what the heck! Anyway, the big deal is that Boyd says that his itching stopped real quick when he put it on. It was the same way with me! Can you believe it? I'll tell ya this much, my mom won't believe it! But man, my headache is gone! Thank you, sir! Thank you, I'm sure glad you're not a lawyer. Hey Mr. Graham, my little brother wants to say hi."

"Hello, Mr. Graham, thank you for puttin' an end to our scratchin'. It sure feels a lot better now."

What a way to go back to sleep. Two boys soaking in a bath of clay, and it working so well! What a payoff for detoxing with Clay Therapy. Too much!

The next day I got the whole story. It didn't take long, and it wasn't a very nice story. When the accident happened, the railroad stonewalled the whole issue. They tried to create the impression that the whole incident was no big deal. The city fathers, afraid the whole thing would cost them tourist dollars, put little effort into alerting the community regarding the seriousness of the situation. The local doctors, who owed their allegiance to the railroad, and who couldn't effectively treat chemical poisoning anyway, maintained that no real problem existed. Other doctors who admitted to the problem said that nothing could be done to alleviate symptoms of the bleeding gums, headaches, rashes, fatigue, skin coming off children's feet, miscarriages, multiple periods for women, aching joints, etc.

All the while, Melvin Belli, the famous attorney from San Francisco, California (since deceased), sent a staff of attorneys to Dunsmuir to set up shop and start the process of acquiring clients for lawsuits against the railroad.

The legal profession is well aware that for all practical purposes, nothing in medicine will satisfactorily alleviate the symptoms of chemical poisoning. By the time I got there, the Belli organization had hired a chemical sensitivity specialist, a toxicologist from the San Fernando Valley in California, Gunnar Heuser, M.D. Dr. Heuser worked as an assistant clinical professor of medicine at the U.C.L.A. School of Medicine. He came to conduct weekly examinations, to document symptoms on many of those who were injured.

As though being led, I started to explain to people in the community, one by one, what I was doing, and offered the clay free to anyone with symptoms. It was inspiring. My clay worked quickly and consistently on men, women, and children. I could predict results, and word quickly spread.

Everyone who used clay for headaches got relief quickly, usually in an hour or two. The rashes disappeared within a day or so, and in all cases, I suggested they continue the treatment daily for several weeks.

As I digested all of this, I was called back to the L.A. area to take care of some serious problems with my side business. Joyce and I stayed with Mom, and when it was time to leave, we decided Joyce would remain there. We knew our situation was hot and things could break open at any time. Joyce stayed behind to make sure Mom didn't have to deal with it.

When I returned to Dunsmuir, I found out where Dr. Heuser was taking the case histories for those injured. He didn't stay in Dunsmuir. Many people wisely wouldn't enter the community at all. Many believed that the toxic particles remained on the trees and grass, and still contaminated the houses of those who lived there.

I might add that Dr. Heuser's name surfaced in a major article written for a national publication, "The Mystery of Multiple Chemical Sensitivity and Gulf War Syndrome: Something in the Air," by Linda Bonvie and Bill Bonvie.

Dr. Heuser, and those working with him, chose to stay and do their work in McCloud, a little community twenty miles from Dunsmuir, and higher up in the mountains.

I soon realized the disaster had attracted other large environmental organizations there, too. The Chemically Injured Hotline people were there, and the Environmentally Sensitive

Group, both national organizations.

I introduced myself and told them that I had reason to believe that using clay to detox would bring a degree of relief to those suffering chemical poisoning. They were, to a person, taken aback and curious. They had no idea that anything could help the detoxification process, or bring relief to those enduring the symptoms.

They told me that people all over the country were being chemically injured, and that nothing seemed to help. Those uninformed about what I'd already done thought I was deluding myself about the capabilities of clay, and that it was laughable for me to believe my clay could affect the suffering of these people.

These well-meaning and caring people couldn't get outside their paradigm to *imagine* that anything would bring any relief. Of course, I had to remember that they didn't come to research remedies, but to document the problem. Some of these activists had been hurt badly by Chemical Poisoning and treated by the most sophisticated methods known to medicine.

I met Dr. Heuser and his lovely wife, a very quiet lady, and I had the impression that she may have known about clay therapy from someplace else, but I never found out for sure. The doctor couldn't imagine that anything could help this problem. He hadn't come to treat people anyway. He had come as a toxicologist hired by the Belli Group to document case histories.

I talked with Dr. Heuser and presented my plan, which he approved. That plan included meeting his clients as they left the hotel to give them the dry and gelled packages of clay along with instructions for its use. I also gave them other information about clay therapy, along with written instructions. I told them to call me if they needed to, I'd see them next week when they returned to see Dr. Heuser for his follow-up.

It seemed the entire population of Dunsmuir was angry and scared, because no one had any idea of the long-term effects. People had heard many stories of other chemical poisonings, and the townspeople were well aware that the doctors didn't have any answers, which frightened them. Soon enough my continued presence force-fed the issue of clay therapy and caused the environmental activists to seriously examine the phenomenon of clay therapy for detox.

Big Dollars

At the same time, the rumors about my clay helping people circulated. Then sadly the lawyers introduced a new ingredient to the toxic soup: big money. Dunsmuir has a lot of hard-working people, and the chance to collect on a big lawsuit was very attractive, albeit a very dangerous form of Russian roulette. Many good people refused my treatment because they thought it might affect their chances to collect from a lawsuit.

One of the first families I saw in McCloud lived close to the river, and they had pronounced and obvious symptoms. When they came by the table I had set up outside, the man said, "Now I know who you are! I've heard about what you're doing. We'll give that stuff to the kids, but it's not for me or the wife."

His wife looked frightened. "Mister, the lawyer said we have a good lawsuit, and we don't want nothin' to ruin it. We've heard about what you did. We'll do it after this legal thing is over, but not now."

I replied, "We don't yet know about the long-term benefits of this treatment, but so far it looks awfully good. Are you sure you want to take such a big chance? It looks to me as if we can stop what might be a big problem developing later in your life."

"I got to, Mister, I just got to. It's big dollars."

I've never felt so sorry for anyone as I did for that couple.

A Dollar is Only Worth A Dollar

A young lawyer and a physician from California examined a client named Robert Bryant for the symptoms of chemical poisoning. Satisfied by the nature of his symptoms, they qualified him for a generous settlement.

The Bryant family, at least Mrs. Bryant and her three children, had been in Portland, Oregon for a funeral two days before, and three days after the fateful night of the chemical spill. However, her husband had two very unlucky events happen to him. He had been chemically injured six years before in Sacramento, and he slept only a hundred feet from the thick cloud of toxic gas.

He was in bad shape, struggling with a blinding headache and a fearsome rash. Fortunately, he had friends who advised him about what I was doing. Lawsuit or not, he'd had enough, and at 7:00 p.m. on September 14, 1991, he called and asked if I would see him, so he could get started on the "stuff." I went to his house, and he started the process. By 9.00 p.m., when I called him, he was much better from the "bitch of a headache."

He had gone through the treatment routine several times, and when his doctor and lawyer paid him a visit twenty-six hours after their original inspection, they were amazed by his progress. After a thorough examination of this big tough mill worker, who had been suffering when last interviewed, they declared him "amazingly clear" relative to his condition the day before.

He had passed up thousands of needed dollars, for his health and the sake of his family.

I called and told him I was on my way over. When I arrived, he pulled his big frame out of the chair, ambled over, tucked his shirt in, stuck out his huge hand, and smiled at me.

He said, "Hell, Cano, a dollar is only worth a dollar."

The evening of the first day at the hotel was interesting. It was a rustic old place. Dr. Heuser and his wife, the Chemically Injured Hotline people, the Environmentally Sensitive Group and their helpers made a very unique group. They had all come to document the physical and emotional effect of the Dunsmuir Spill. I came to prove what clay could do for detoxification and to assist the healing process from chemical poisoning.

What a group. I have always admired activists, and those who work to solve such problems have got my vote. Many of them had been injured by chemical exposure, so they vigorously worked to expose the problem.

That evening, the conversation drifted to different aspects of the problem, from the transportation of these deadly chemicals, to accidents, to those responsible, to the reaction of the Dunsmuir officials and local doctors. Then the conversation turned to the symptoms and the case histories for the upcoming lawsuits.

However, as the evening stretched on, the more obvious it became that my presence created an awkward situation and everyone tried to avoid the concept that anything could be done to treat those who were injured. Their *head in the sand* approach fascinated me, although two of the women doing the testing had first-hand experience with what I was doing. They were all in the business of gathering data, and not interested in solving the health problem.

Finally, Dr. Heuser led the conversation around to me, and my interest in detoxing and treating chemical poisoning.

The doctor's curiosity led others to ask questions. They could no longer ignore the reality of clay therapy. Everyone treated me with politeness, but they were just patronizing me.

The questions they didn't ask began to unravel their shroud. The questions they did ask were well intentioned but shallow. The next morning, a call came in for me.

A lady on the other end said, "Mr. Graham? This is Betty Reed. I met you with my two daughters yesterday?"

"Oh, yes."

She said, "Well, I *am* surprised! You said not to be surprised if there were observable results by the following day, and sure enough it happened. You didn't meet my husband, but he said, 'To hell with the lawsuit. It might be years before they come through, and this headache is killing me. Let me try that stuff.' It worked for all of us. It's a miracle! We want you to come by and have dinner with us. Will you?"

Tears came to my eyes.

An hour later, another family called to tell Dr. Heuser a similar story. He was astonished. I was elated!

The people in the hotel lobby all stood around having various conversations. The doctor waved to me and pulled me aside. "This is all very interesting, but I came here to document symptoms, not to treat patients."

"Doc, it might be interesting to you folks, but it's a miracle to those who had no option yesterday. Our system is unbelievable. You've never even been afforded the opportunity to read about the subject of clay therapy, have you, Doctor?"

He immediately retreated to his tower. "There are many remedies for various problems that I don't pay much attention to."

"Be that as it may, we both seem to have learned a lot in the past 24 hours." He sounded puzzled. "Is it used for anything else?"

I loved it! "Oh, yes. Many things, both external and internal."

"Really?" Then he made a statement that I'll never forget. He said, in his very proper, and sophisticated German accent, "You know, Mr. Graham, I never trust any medication that works for more than one purpose."

"Oh, really? Doc, we've already stopped headaches and rashes. That's two and still working. You're a toxicologist, right? Do you have other medical interests?"

"Yes, I do. I have a practice that deals with migraine headaches."

"You do?" I followed up with, "Aren't they treated several ways? Doc, Doc, Doc. We have a lot to talk about. First, I heard you mention shingles last night, and how it's a very tough condition to treat? Doc, you just ain't gonna believe just how fast this lady will go to work on shingles, and that's just for openers!"

"What lady?"

"Excuse me, it's simply how I refer to her...the clay. We have a lot of things to discuss." I was in heaven.

One of the most highly visible attorneys in the country had a respected toxicologist documenting the symptoms of those injured by an internationally exposed (news-wise), chemical poisoning of major proportions, and many were now using clay therapy and getting very positive results. Yes! Literally, my prayers were being answered. My lady was going to have her day! All I needed was a little more time.

That evening, however, the second shoe finally fell. That night I called mom to tell her how things were going in Dunsmuir, and to ask how she was feeling. She had a slight numbness in her right arm, but all in all she was doing great.

"Joyce and I are doing fine." She said.

Music to my ears. She's happy and well. "Great, Mom. Listen, let me talk to Joyce. I'm so glad things are going well."

"Sure, just a minute. Joyce! Cano wants to talk to you. She'll be right here. It's so good to hear the news up there. Here she is." Mom sounded wonderful.

"Hi, Cano."

"Hi, gal. How's mom doing, really?"

She's doing terrific. I just taught her how to make cornbread West Texas style. She's hard to keep up with. Eva's amazing."

"That's a natural fact."

"But Cano, listen. Eva just went to the bathroom, and there's something I've got to tell you. I'm so glad you called."

"What's up?"

"Cano, the U.S. Marshals came by. They want to talk to you, that's what they said. They left a card and want you to call 'em."

"Does mother know about this?"

"No, she was asleep. She has no idea.."

"Joyce, It's all coming down. I'll keep you posted. Do they know I'm here?"

"I don't think so, but some of the neighbors know, so I'm not sure."

"Thanks for being so cool about all this. I'll call you tomorrow." It was October 15, 1991. I had to leave Dunsmuir that evening. I couldn't risk staying another night.

I never had dinner with Mr. and Mrs. Reed and their two lovely daughters. I never got to see Nick and Boyd again. I had to return to Southern California, via San Francisco, and face a very different life. I had finally run out of time.

⚃ ⚃ ⚃

The Dunsmuir Spill was more of a disaster than originally thought, and more fish and animals were affected than estimated at the time. Some species became extinct. Experts have told us the ecosystem will take fifty years to recover.

And what about the people? Only time will tell. Many remain bitter over the final results, and many lives have been scarred forever by the disaster at Dunsmuir. Some call it a tough break. Many gambled. Some lost big, and some won, but got no money.

It's happened before, and it will happen again.

The use of pesticides and herbicides, along with the by-products of American Industry, sets the stage for a horrible payback for our progress and our avarice. Rachel Carson gave us fair warning in *The Silent Spring* fifty years ago. We Clay Disciples give you a promise: These are the old times. Learn how clay therapy can help you and your grandchildren's grandchildren survive. The Power created clay for the benefit of all living things.

⚃ ⚃ ⚃

During the time in Dunsmuir, I also took periodic trips to San Francisco in an attempt to introduce clay to people who were HIV positive, and to those with AIDS. This surreal attempt was my last-ditch effort to authenticate, in a highly visible manner, the validity of my clay in the therapeutic treatment of AIDS victims, and it grew into an obsession. I figured if I could just get Clay Therapy recognized as an adjunct to AIDS therapy, my clay's integrity would carry it the rest of the way.

A man in Dunsmuir, California, told me of a friend who had AIDS in San Francisco, and someone else in Sonora, California, told me of someone they knew. Both lived in the San Francisco area. I headed for San Francisco with my clay when I left Dunsmuir.

At the time, although I knew a great deal about Clay Therapy I hadn't slowed up enough to write down any of my experiences with its usage. I had no record of clay therapy's ability to help a lot of the problems that plagued many AIDS victims. I knew what Clay Therapy could do, I just needed time to prove that it could effectively treat many of the symptoms, or at least offer some relief.

When I first arrived in San Francisco, it struck me as so busy and confusing that I thought I would never get oriented. I knew I'd need help in reaching the people I felt I could help, so I first sought out an organization that distributed hundreds of meals to AIDS victims at their homes. I caught up with the woman who headed the project, a dedicated professional. I found her in the loading area while she issued orders and checked her clipboard for details.

"Hi, I'm Cano Graham. I have the largest pure Therapeutic Clay Center in the country. I believe that I can be of service to the AIDS community."

"Clay?" She blinked.

For just a moment I thought that maybe she knew about Clay Therapy. I said, "I've prepared close to a thousand sacks of dry and gelled clay, along with instructions for its use. I could talk to your drivers and teach them about its value, and how to use it, or I could ride with them and talk to each patient personally. I'd be more than glad to work anyway you wish." This would be the mother lode for research and results!

"Tell me more, Mr. Graham," she said.

I handed her the sheet of instructions I had prepared. "Ma'am, I've written these instructions specifically for HIV/AIDS victims.

As you can see, I've outlined many applications. I start with the full range of topical applications for the sores, the rashes, the infections, as well as for the ones that wouldn't heal, you know, the fungus stuff, the yeast infections, the mouth sores, the dental decay, and the general deterioration of the oral tissues that make it almost impossible for AIDS victims to eat."

Her interest excited me. I might get to help hundreds, maybe thousands.

I continued. "In addition, they could detoxify their systems and start pulling waste from their tissues by immersing themselves in a full-body clay bath! We have unlimited possibilities here."

I took care to tone down my enthusiasm a bit. I didn't want her to see me as a maniac babbling on and on about 'dirt' of some kind. I never suggested that the clay could stop or cure the AIDS virus. I only wanted to help prove clay would alleviate much of the suffering AIDS caused.

She rubbed her forehead with one hand and held her clipboard in the other. She glanced up at me and squinted. "Mr. Graham, we have many people who want to help, but we simply deliver food to AIDS victims. I'm sure you don't want us to feed them clay, do you? Thanks for your interest." She closed the scene by sticking out her hand for me to shake.

All of a sudden it seemed cooler. Something was wrong with this picture. The light had a different hue, and everyone just went right on busily doing his or her job. I decided to implement plan B and headed for Oakland, California.

Joyce's friends in Sonora told us of a man in Oakland with AIDS. James, an African-American, had a T-cell count of 250. After proper introductions, I gave him a book to read about Clay Therapy, and he said he'd read the book and talk to his doctor, a woman who specialized in the treatment of AIDS. After James read the book, he expressed a polite curiosity, but he said that his doctor had blown up at the mention of something as unconventional as Clay Therapy to treat AIDS victims. She considered it a total waste of time, and absolutely insane to even consider such a bizarre treatment option.

Well, I figured, you can't win 'em all, but I had to think of some way to crack the issue open and break through the wall of medical skepticism. I read the gay newspapers, trying to find some individual who was researching new methods and ideas. I frantically made calls to different groups. The main problem was that I didn't know my way around. Time became my worst enemy, and it was a commodity that I was almost out of! The weather grew cooler, and the thought of November's approach was like a long winter shadow growing shorter, and shorter.

I went to see a gentleman by the name of Bryan who had been recommended to me by a man in Dunsmuir. I found his apartment up a flight of stairs, off Mission Street. From the first moment I met Bryan, he made me feel comfortable. We talked about small stuff, and he soon realized that I had never, to my knowledge, seen anyone with AIDS.

"I'm your first?"

"Yeah. I think so...well...sort of. I didn't get too far with a guy in Oakland I met. His doctor shut me off."

"I can understand that," he said smiling. "Randy in Dunsmuir says you've done a remarkable thing with that chemical poisoning in the Sacramento River. He said that many people there are totally dumbfounded by what you've done with your clay."

"Yes, thanks, it's really been one hell of an experience, very gratifying."

"You seem to be covering a lot of ground. Who are you?"

I told him about my Therapeutic Clay Center in the desert and about the clay. I further discussed what I thought of using clay as a fundamental therapy to treat the symptoms of AIDS, and wound up by saying, "So, that's the broad strokes on what clay therapy is about. "The problem is that I'm running out of time!"

He snickered and said, "Aren't we all!"

"Yes, I see your point. You're up against it in one way, and

I'm up against it in another. Bryan, just so you'll understand: I'll soon be indicted and sent to Federal Prison, soon, real soon."

"Why don't you split?"

"It doesn't fit."

"Okay, very, very interesting. Cano, have you ever seen a melosarcomic type of cancer, or what it does to its victims?"

"No, I haven't, but I'd like to."

"Too bad you can't hang around town." Then he laughed, and said like Jimmy Durante, "We got a million of 'em." Then he pointed to a bruise-like spot on his leg. "There's one right there."

"What are those spots there?" I pointed to a group of sores.

"Just sores. They heal slowly or not at all."

"Have you got bleeding gums?" I questioned him further.

"I've got the whole nine yards of AIDS symptoms!" He retorted. "I'm sick, Cano. I'm sicker that you know. I mean, right now I am so sick…"

I could see, hear, and feel his pain. "I'm sorry, Bryan. So very, very sorry." I said, getting up to go. "I've got to leave for L.A. May I call you in a few days?"

"Sure, Cano, give me a call."

"Thanks. Now then, I'm going to leave a lot of my clay with you, and I truly hope you'll use it yourself, and spread it around to others."

"I'll sure do my best." Bryan smiled bravely. He had the look of November in his thin face.

"Cano, did you see a bottle of water at the foot of the stairs?"

"Yes. Can I get it for you?"

"Would you be so kind?"

I got the water, and was placing it on the dispenser, when I said, "This was an important day for me, to be able to see and visit with you and all. Thanks so very much!"

Then he said, "These days *are* precious, aren't they?"

At that moment I felt a cold jolt through my body. "Why'd you say that?"

"What?" he asked.

"Precious, you mentioned precious days."

"They just are." He replied with a shrug. "They simply are very precious days." I gave him a big hug. He hugged me back. "I wish you were going to be around. I think you would and could do a lot of good in our town."

"Thanks. Thanks so very much for those words, Bryan. I really wish I could, but, I'm running out of options," and I let it drop at that.

The days dwindled to a precious few. I called Bryan four days later just as I was leaving San Francisco, and a friend of his answered the phone. When I asked if Bryan was there, he said, "Bryan is very sick right now. Is this Cano, the clay man?"

"Yes, it is."

"Hi, Cano. I know everyone who would normally call, and I didn't recognize your voice. Bryan wanted me to tell you that your clay was working on his sores! Several of us are using it. Thanks so much. Bryan knew you'd be glad to hear the news."

The day was bright, crisp, and very San Fransisco-ish. It was October 25, 1991.

"Thank you so very much. Tell Bryan that he made my day!"

Chapter 40

September's Song

Everything is only for a day, both that which remembers and that which is remembered. Marcus Aurelius

As the end neared, a melancholy suffused me, and the haunting lyrics of "September's Song" went round and round in my head.

And the days dwindle down to a precious few
September, November,
And these few precious days,
I'll spend with you.

Depression drifted like an unwanted fog into my being, coloring my emotions just as the golden leaves covered the brown grass. The hint of 1991's fall crispness in the breeze sadly replaced the smells of summer. My world was imploding, and the relentless pressure squeezing my mind was like a cheap rendition of the Chinese water torture. The sands of time were running out for me, and I was keenly aware that any hour could be my last hour of freedom. I knew with a certainty that indictment and Federal Prison awaited me.

The government had already seized all of my property in Tecopa Hot Springs, crushing all my dreams for our Healing Community, and I knew of no one willing to step in and take my place.

I have no happy ending to this sad chapter. I have no interesting stories to relate, and no good times to share. My world began to collapse. Mother had a massive stroke, and besides other complications, it left her paralyzed on her right side.

My mother was down, not getting up, and I would soon go to Federal Prison. But now, considering this news about mom, my future simply didn't matter anymore. I steeled myself to face my Armageddon. Under normal circumstances, I'd drive like a madman to her bedside, but I didn't. A couple of hours or so either way wouldn't make any difference at this stage.

I got the news from Joyce around 3 p.m. I knew it would be too late to see mom that night since I had an eight to ten hour drive from San Francisco. In fact I drove slower than usual down the coast of California on famous 101 and arrived at a motel in Chino not far from the Chino hospital where Mother lay.

I didn't want to stay at Mother's for fear the Federal Marshals might take me in before I had everything done that needed doing. I'd go voluntarily in a week or so. Several 'Biz' friends deserved assurance that when I fell I would fall alone. And I had a list of others I simply wanted to say good-bye to. But tonight, I would rest. It was two a.m.

God gave us memory so that we might have roses in December.
James M. Barrie

Chapter 41

Strangers In The Night

Man loves company even if that of only a small burning candle.
Georg Christoph Lichtenberg

I looked out my motel window and saw a cold rain, driven by a gusty wind. Like I needed more of this weather to seal my mood. Although tired, I was also hungry and needed to relax so I could sleep. I decided to throw a coat on and walked a block for a bowl of chili. A hot bowl of chili with crackers sometimes works, when nothing else will. The chili was good, but my mood remained, like the after effect of a bad dream.

When I returned to my second floor room, which faced the street, the busy sounds of the traffic below, and the lights of the city flashing at me put me on edge. I had the idea of getting out of the biting wind and rain, and finding a dark, quiet sheltered place outside to mull over some things. I walked around on the balcony to the backside of the motel where, besides being out of the wind and rain, I found a tranquil view overlooking a vacant field and a row of homes.

Before long I drifted into an old habit of wondering what's going on in a particular house. Who's there? What do they do? What are they dealing with as I stand here? Then my thoughts drifted back to my present situation, and the possibilities for the future, a future that contained only abstract images. For some strange reason I flashed on a children's merry-go-round, with the ponies and lions going up and down, and 'round and 'round, headed nowhere.

Then I thought about my lawyer, who was first a so called

friend, and who had taken many, many thousands of dollars from me, at first by conning me into believing that he could really help me, and then keeping me terrified for months by telling me that my arrest was imminent. I wondered if he was cozily sitting at home.

After about a half hour, I realized that the weather had turned colder, and I shivered in the self-imposed exile of my mind. I was no closer to a solution than I had been before leaving for the diner, and my current dreamlike state of mind was only a temporary escape from the reality of my situation. I knew I'd only find relief with a few hours of blissfully unaware sleep.

Suddenly, a gust of wind snapped me around, and I chanced to glance down the stairs leading to the first floor because I thought I heard a cat.

Meeeoowwww.

I heard it again, that plaintive sound that a cat makes when he wants something.

Then I finally saw him, a big tomcat with black and white splashes, soaking wet, and miserable looking. I wondered what he was doing out in this weather. He looked straight up at me and cried out again. I didn't need a wet cat, and I guessed he belonged to someone who lived close by. The cat cried out again, more loudly this time.

He looked up at me and shook his left paw.

"Sorry pal, you'd better go on home. A little rain won't hurt you, and someone is probably worried about you."

He cried out again, looking up directly at me, waving his paw the way cats do when they're wet, or hurt. Then he got serious. He came up the steps towards me. As I turned away, he let out a scary scream.

"What the hell do you want?" I spoke to him as if he were a person. "What's up? Is something the matter? What's wrong with you?"

He shook his paw at me and meowed like crazy, and it sort of spooked me. This cat was not only talking to me, but was seriously trying to get my attention.

"Okay, you've got something to say?" Well, what is it? You want something right?" I began to descend the stairs.

He sat down on one of the steps, looked at me and shook his paw.

"What've you got there, a sticker? What's the tape for?"

Meowww!

That cat seemed sure I had an answer for his problem, whatever it was. What the hell. I decided to get busy, wet cat and all. I was right on target. He had a collar, and I got the impression that he lived in the neighborhood. Then again, maybe he had escaped from someone's car.

Anyway, we talked it over for a few seconds, and I sat down beside him. He started the old rubbing routine, so I lifted him onto my lap. It didn't take a brain surgeon to figure out what had happened to him. He had cut his paw or been in a fight, and some kid, or fool of more advanced age had put tape around the wound. It was infected, swollen and septic. No wonder he was crying for help! It was driving him crazy!

"Okay, pal, this is a cinch. I'm going to take you upstairs right now, and put some clay on your paw, and then I'll clip the tape off. So that's it. Are you ready?"

I took him upstairs to my room, and gently rubbed clay around the affected area before clipping away the tape. Doing it that way, reduced the pain and made the tape come off easier when cut.

I gave him some of the tuna I carried for a snack and allowed him to stay the night, but that was it! I explained to him that he'd have to sleep on the floor because that is where a cat belonged. He slept on the bed, close to my backside.

The next morning, I checked out of the motel. I had some running around to do after I saw mom and might be gone for the night. Before leaving, I put more clay on the tom cat's paw and turned him loose.

The Last Days

Live all you can; it's a mistake not to. It doesn't so much matter what you do in particular, so long as you have your life. If you haven't had that, what have you had?   Henry James

When I arrived at the hospital, I found a doctor and two nurses standing in the hallway.

I recognized one of the nurses. "Hi, Mr. Graham, this is Dr. John Reed."

"Hello, Mrs. Parker, good to see you here. Doctor, it's nice to meet you." We shook hands.

"Mr. Graham, I'll be your mother's physician through this episode. I haven't met you in the flesh, but I understand you and your mother are well known to the staff around Chino General, and your mother seems to be a favorite."

"Thanks Doctor, she's everybody's favorite. And please call me, Cano. Doc, how is she?"

"Cano, she's bouncing back in strong fashion. She had a tough go of it, but as you well know, your mom has an amazing constitution. She had a stroke in her left temporal lobe causing her right side to be affected, but we feel with medication and physical therapy she'll continue to come around. I might also say that she's certainly improving. Of course that's not to say we're completely out of the woods. The next seventy-two hours will tell us a lot."

"I realize this is a difficult question but, how does it look in general? What's the prognosis? Please be candid with me."

"Cano, your mom's tired. The last operation took a lot out of her. God knows she's brave, but she's tired. Her body's fragile, and she needs a lot of rest. I'm glad you're here. Her speech has been affected but the nurses say she's been calling for you."

"Doctor, will she walk out of here?"

"It's simply too soon to tell, but if courage has anything to do with it, she will. At her age, and with the seriousness of the

317

damage, well, it's hard to say. But rest assured that we've had great results with our treatment plan in these cases. First, she needs a lot of rest."

Doctor Reed had put his remarks in a most intelligent, straightforward, and compassionate way. I appreciated his words and liked the man, but mom was down. Eighty-nine years of constant action had taken its toll. Her body had finally worn out. She had no reserves left. She operated on courage alone.

I found a neighbor and good friend, Ethel Williamson, sitting with mom. She put her finger to her lips to indicate mom was sleeping. We left the room, and embraced the way friends do when they're giving and seeking support in times of shared grief.

Ethel said, "I'm so relieved you're here. Joyce called me as soon as it happened, and also told me you were on the way. Dear, it's difficult to understand Eva, but she's been calling for you. She's in and out of sleep. I think she's dreaming. Oh, I'm so glad you're here. Are you all right?"

"Yes, I'm fine. I slept well last night. I got in late, too late to come here. What do you think? Will she make it?"

"Cano, we almost lost her. If it hadn't been for Joyce, I think we would have. She reacted like a veteran. She knew exactly what to do. I mean she instantly called 911 and proceeded to keep her head raised until the EMTs got there.

"Joyce is a special one."

"Dear, Eva is so weak, also her speech is slurred. We can't understand her too well, but maybe you will. But anyway she'll be so happy to see you. Before we see her I've got to ask, when do you go in?"

"I figure about a week. Hey, mom doesn't know?"

"No! The few of us who know have kept it from her, not a hint."

"Good. I've got so much to do. I'll be with her everyday, but I've got a lot of driving to do. I'll be staying in town, and then come back here in the day. I've got to close some things down.

You know, things I should do and friends I want to see."

Ethel took my hand. "I understand. Dear, I'll leave you and Eva alone. She'll wake up soon."

"Thanks Ethel, it means a lot to know you can be with her."

I had a hunch mom could faintly hear our voices in the hall, and I was right. When I entered her room she turned her head in my direction. I bent over, held my face to her cheek, and kissed away a tear. She knew I was there. We stayed that way for several minutes. I pulled a chair up close so I could lean on the bed near her.

I held her left hand, and whispered, "Hi, Honey. I know you can hear me and I know you're thinking. You understand me. Right?"

She slightly nodded yes, and squeezed my hand twice. "Doctor Reed says you're doing real good, and responding to their treatments. Hey, Honey, you're popular around here. Nurse Parker told me several of the aids want to care for you. Maria especially. They all love ya. I understand Joyce did a wonderful job when this happened."

She squeezed my hand tightly several times in a row. Then Mom kinda pulled me close and tried to say something. I got close to her and then I understood.

"You want to know about Dunsmuir?"

She squeezed my hand twice. "Okay I got it. Two means yes?"

She squeezed again twice. Mom never failed to amaze me. Here she was in a life-threatening position, and was really interested in my work at the Dunsmuir Spill. Plus she had already devised a way to communicate. She was thinking. Was Eva Graham something else or what?

"Honey, I'm so fortunate that you encouraged me to go. I mean things went better than I ever expected, much better because the results were documented by a specialist."

Mom squeezed my hand rapidly. I knew she wanted details.

"Honey, people had bad headaches, rashes all over their

bodies. They had sores and bleeding gums, and some women were even having multiple periods. They were all screwed up. It was something. Lawyers were there from San Francisco lining up lawsuits for those injured. I found that a real problem with this chemical injury stuff is that the doctors don't have anyway to treat it. I assumed they did, and they don't. Can you believe it?"

Mom tried to say something. I leaned closer. She slurred, "Terrible!"

"Mom our clay worked! And quick. I wish you could have been there. The headaches were gone in an hour or so. Gone! And these people have had 'em since the accident happened. Rashes were the best part for me for two reasons; one was everyone had 'em bad, and you could see 'em so when they cleared up in a day or two everyone knew, and was talking. It was incredible. I had no idea the clay would work so fast on that kind of thing. There are a lot of people suffering with the effects of these toxins. I mean all over the country."

Mom turned her head, looked at me and started squeezing my hand steadily. She loved the report and knew its significance. I kissed her. She looked at me and through those tired but still expressive eyes smiled and seemed contented.

Maria came into the room with a tray. "Hi, Cano, I heard you were here. Would you care for some coffee and a pastry? It's *pan dulce*, you know Mexican sweet bread."

"Hello, María! Mom, it's María. I'm so glad you're here. Wonderful to see you, yes I'd love it. Thanks so much."

"Oh, *de nada*, I'm happy to do it. How's our girl?"

"She's doing well, she has a way to go, but she'll get there."

"We'll take good care of her."

"I know you will, and you probably already know this, but mother can understand what we're saying easy enough. She just can't talk too well."

"Yes, I know."

"But if you want to ask her questions just hold her left hand the way I'm doing, and she can give you one squeeze for no and two for yes, or you guys can work it out."

Mom squeezed my hand twice firmly. She liked the idea of running her own show and playing the hand she was dealt.

Maria had other work to do and said, "I got to go, glad you're here-bye." And then, "Oh I almost forgot. Cano, your clay is a real big hit in my neighborhood."

"Thanks, Maria, a lot." She left the room and I got close to mom. "Are you sleepy?"

She instantly squeezed my hand with one long hard nooo! She wanted to talk. She wanted us together. I'd soon be gone, and never hold her hand or see her face again. I desperately tried to control my emotions.

I reversed gears, "Honey, I've got good news and bad news. The good news is, you remember I told you about the Clay business and fishing trip I was invited to with my old army buddies. Remember?"

She squeezed my hand twice.

"Well, I talked to my old friend, told him about Dunsmuir, and he seems to think I could get a lot done with our clay because so many workers there suffer with the effects of herbicides and pesticides." I tried my best to create a story that would make sense to her. It was hard to fool mother.

"It looks like a real opportunity, but it'll take some time, maybe a month or so, and I sure don't want to be gone that long."

She pulled me near and through a slurred whisper said, "Go, honey, go!"

"But it could be a month-maybe longer."

She pulled my hand again, looked deeply into my eyes, and whispered, "Please go. Do it for momma. Go do what you do. I'll be fine. Maybe there's others like Dunsmuir."

This tore me up, but it was her way. She would actually get more satisfaction, more sense of accomplishment for herself, if she encouraged me to go rather than if I stayed. She had been with me every step along the way, and she'd be with me there in her mind. Mom understood the clay's worth, and my dreams. She also thought fishing was the best recreation, besides dancing, one could enjoy, and that I should do more of it. What she loved most was what she wanted for me.

"All right, honey. It'll be a week or so before I leave, and I've got a zillion things to do. I'll be here in the morning and spend all day."

She squeezed twice. Mom turned her head and winked.

"Also Joyce is taking care of everything perfectly, so we're in good shape at home."

I spent everyday with mom, and at night I'd hit the road seeing friends while wrapping things up. Each day I left was more excruciating than the day before. I was driving back to the Chino Motel. It was November 4th, 1991. I was seriously near being incapacitated. I couldn't focus on driving. Mother wasn't responding as I had hoped. The curtain was coming down. I had accepted going to prison, though I didn't know for how long. But with mom struggling so, everything changed. I now faced the fact that unless I pulled a very short sentence, which by now I knew unlikely, or found not guilty, totally out of the question, tomorrow could well be the last day I'd ever see her again.

The thought was paralyzing. I became physically sick with a maddening despair and found myself coming to a stop in the parking lot of the Chino Motel at around 10:30 p.m. The next morning would be my last with Mother. I had only a few more hours with her; a few hours after a full life together as mother and son. My world was coming to an end. I was only hours away.

Before I checked out I had a call to make. I called Bryan in San Francisco. His friend answered and told me that Bryan had unexpectedly died last night, Nov. 4th. Then I made my way to the hospital. When I walked into mother's room, bent over, kissed her, and took her hand, she turned to me and through her difficult speech observed, "What's wrong honey? You don't look well."

I didn't want to talk much for fear of losing it. I had to concentrate to hold my poise when I said lightheartedly, "Ah, Gal I just don't want to leave you."

I had to get closer to understand her. She seemed weaker.

She looked at me and said, "Honey, don't say that. Please, it would make momma feel terrible if you missed this. Please go. Do your work and have fun. When you get back I'll be at home with Joyce, and it'll be like always. I'll miss you, and I can't wait to see you again."

With that said, I caved in and rested my tearful face on her pillow. She brought her left hand up and stroked my hair and face. She whispered softly, "Send me some pictures, and write to me. Would you? I'd love to know what you're seeing and doing." She was very tired.

"Honey, momma's sleepy now. Would you rub my toes?" And she closed her eyes.

I started to brush her toes with my fingertips, when she smiled slightly, and fell sound asleep.

Maria entered the room. "She loves that so much."

I turned to Maria, "Yes, yes she does. Please do it often, Maria. And would you please excuse me, I'd like to be alone with mom for a while. I won't be here for sometime. I'm going out of state."

I don't recall leaving the hospital, nor being driven to the U.S. Marshall's. It was November 5, 1991. The precious days were over.

Chapter 42

County Jail

Adapt or perish, now as ever, is Nature's inexorable imperative.
H. G. Wells

I awaited trial for eight months, housed in Midwestern County jails that held anywhere from 50 to 250 prisoners. The population of these places changes often, but always there were a few local characters, several smart-ass punks with their first tattoos, and a mixed bag of street corner crack dealers. All the rest were continually subjected to a morning dose of cartoons, with the sound cranked up full blast so they could be heard above the asinine domino players 'slamming' on steel tables. Which, by the way, sounded remarkably like either being underneath a steel table when someone was striking it with a small ball peen hammer, or the shrill ping of a .22 rifle next to your ear.

In each cellblock, above all the incessant noise you could always hear two or three obscene loud mouths trying to outtalk each other over a no-brainer issue, and not with logic, but by sheer posturing, and volume.

The cumulative effect of these, and other more physically dangerous factors, coupled with not knowing how long or when it would ever end, created an emotional slaughterhouse. Despite the supposed moderate temperature in the cellblock, I was constantly cold, a reflection of the winter temperatures outside.

Sleep came fitfully and painfully on a light blue solid concrete bunk, with only a pitifully thin, cracked plastic pad for a mattress. I rested my head on a pillow, an inch-thick block made from the same cheap, cold, hard, rotten plastic, and my linens consisted of one blanket, and a towel. An offensive fluorescent tube graced the ceiling, and its cold clammy gray light constantly illuminated my cell.

Lots of pork and no salad or fresh vegetables caused my system to lock up badly. The jailers, a thoughtful group of good ole boys, sold us all the cookies and candy we wanted. The profit went for some police officers fund or whatever.

Besides these terrible conditions, Lucia Solomon and Ethel Williamson informed me that Mother had not continued to improve. They also told me several times - I suppose to make me feel needed and that I hadn't been forgotten - that mom was often calling out at night for me. I couldn't help but think about her doing that. The result had a poisonous effect on my attitude. I heard her echoes in my sleep and sank deeper into a desperate blinding haze of depression.

From the start, my only relief came from writing weekly letters to Mom describing my *Vacation*.

Dec. 17, 1991
Cedar Rapids

Hi, Honey,

For the first time in many years we won't be together for Xmas. This year I'm learning that distance apart has little to do with being together or not, because in many ways I feel closer to you this year than ever before.

I've never felt so near you as when I sense you're having a tough day. I've never felt more joy than those wonderful times when I know you're enjoying a moment special to you - no matter if you're alone or not.

325

I feel a special pride and comfort when those moments come to me that some would call adversity. I reflect on just how you would handle a similar emotion or situation. I know the real blessing of my life was to have a father and mother with the ability to create and enjoy this life. It is a better world because you are here. So, although we can't be together this Xmas maybe this is just God's way of showing us that the love we share for each other is more than strong enough to bridge a little distance. Tonight as every night I start my prayers asking for you to enjoy a good night and awake with that beautiful smile of yours.

I love you so very much
Your proud son,
xx
Cano

In February, they moved me to a small rural county jail where I had a one-man cell, and waited for trial. Same game. Different faces.

February 10, 1992
Vinton, Iowa

Hi, Honey,
    Last night I woke up because this light was on and before I could get back to sleep I found myself smiling to myself because I just knew that at that exact moment you were thinking about me so strong - it was night before last. Do you remember? I almost had the feeling that it was you that woke me up - just by thinking about me. Do you ever do that? It must have been 1:00 at night! Do it again sometime if you find yourself awake - I'll keep a ledger when I get the feeling that you're 'beaming' in on me! - then we can compare notes. I moved from Cedar Rapids to a nice little town called Vinton (5,000 people). I had a good letter from Frank. It

seems his interest in clay is picking up a lot. In fact we're sort of working together on a clay project so you can go to sleep tonight knowing that Frank and I are getting along much better. I know that will make you happy. I miss you so. I miss talking things over with you. Keep thinking about me and try to "beam" in on me. You'll get through!

Love ya,
Cano

March 16, 1992

Dear Mother,

It's a cold and rainy day here, and the forecast says a heavy snow is expected later tonight. Usually this sort of day puts me in the dumps a bit, but I'm really enjoying being here alone. I'm staying in an old friend's one room cabin on a pretty lake that they say is great for fishing. It's one big room, neatly furnished, with a rock fireplace, and overlooking the lake. I do wish you were here.

You know, Mom, I've been thinking about something that led to us, to you and me. You as you, and me as me. You as my mother and me as your son. It's all about the fact that we've been waiting a long time to get here and be mother and son. Last night I had the fire going strong, and was sitting in this big soft chair just looking at the fire. I was thinking of you and Dad, and all of your relatives on each side. I know both sets of grandparents, but I started imaging back past them, way back on both sides.

I mean past your parents and their parent's parents, and back and still further back. The longer I stared at the fire, the further back I could imagine. It was fun wondering who they were, and what they were like.

Honey, there's been many a young man and woman who've fallen in love together, for the past few thousand years, in order for you and Dad to find each other and 'plan' me. By the time I fell asleep the content of the whole evening had caused me to become acutely aware of the precious little time we have together as mother and son.

When the fire had burned down and turned to a bed of coals I found myself focusing on a thought I usually avoid. I couldn't shake the realization of how much time I've wasted, and how much more I could have created with the gifts you blessed me with. I've always been lucky, but the biggest break of my life was without doubt being your third son.

The single finest compliment I will ever be paid was when I heard someone say 'Cano is so like his mother'. I know you heard it too. My last day on earth will be spent remembering, missing, and loving you. Well Sweetheart, I must get some warm clothes on and get ready for my friends.

By the way, I know we've got a long way to go, but if you come back as that big oak tree (which you wanted to be), well–I would gladly be one of your limbs, and stay with you for as long as you stand.

Rest easy
All my love,
Your son~
Cano

Later that same day as I ate a bowl of soup in my cell, the rotund sheriff, with keys jangling plodded slowly to my cell and said, "Graham?"

I didn't look up, and kept spooning my soup.

He coughed and said, "Graham, your mother has died."

I didn't look up and continued to spoon my soup.

He shifted his loose fat frame. "Are you okay?" Then he cleared his throat. "Sorry." He waddled away with his king size key ring keeping perfect time with those laborious steps.

I continued uninterrupted to consume my soup, one spoonful

at a time. The time was about 6:30 p.m. and getting dark. I set my bowl on the small table, and approached the barred windows when I noticed butterfly size snowflakes starting to fall. I folded my arms on the windowsill to watch the small town traffic heading home.

I couldn't imagine or accept this world without her. I laid my head on my arms and wept. I saw the snow fall deep that night.

ෆ ෆ ෆ

Editor's Note: Dr. Frank Graham read Cano's last letter at their mother's funeral on March 19, 1992. Coincidently, considering the Central Standard and Pacific time difference (two hours), Cano wrote this last letter to his mother at almost the exact time on the same morning of her passing.

At the conclusion of Dr. Graham reading his brother's letter, the minister returned to address the congregation. "I have an envelope that was handed to me with these words on the outside: 'Do Not Open. Give this to the minister to read at my funeral. Mom.' I am the one that opened this letter just a little while ago. I would like to read what she has written upon this page."

For my Sons,

When I am gone, cry for me a little, and think of me sometimes, but not too much. It's not good to allow your thoughts to constantly dwell on those who have passed. It is all right to remember some of those special moments but for now you must let me go, and live your lives. You are alive, so let your thoughts be with the living.

All my love forever, Mom

The minister added, "As was always her custom when she wrote her children, Eva Graham signed her name Mom and drew a happy face."

Cano was not aware of his mother's last note until February 2002 when a misplaced tape of the funeral surfaced.

Chapter 43

Day One in Federal Prison

Trust thyself: every heart vibrates to that iron string. Accept the place of divine providence has found for you, the society of your contemporaries, the connection of events.

Ralph Waldo Emerson

The first night I stepped into the plush compound at the Federal Prison in Sheridan, Oregon the clear bright moon suffusing the compound truly astonished me. It had been eight long months since I was last privileged to sit in this audience. Aesthetics aside, this was also a serious Federal Prison, housing an interesting mixture of men, many of which were frankly remarkably similar to those in any decent neighborhood. And yet for one good reason or another the Federal Government had placed them behind sparkling razor wire. I muttered to myself, "Damn, so much natural beauty overseeing such an abundance of pain."

My moon-induced stupor was fractured by an inmate's voice from the Sheridan compound. "These Oregon moons are special, huh?"

Glancing over my shoulder I reacted, "Oh, excuse me, what?" I dropped my duffle bag.

He stepped to my side and said, "Howdy" Then he pointed to the sky. "The moon, you've been watching it for ten minutes! Just drive up?"

"Yeah, for sure the moon is something else. Brings back some old times. Yes, just arrived, but they flew me all over before we landed in Portland."

He laughed at my naive response. "Yes, well, been in county jail right?"

I chuckled, realizing I was so obvious. "You read minds?"

"It's easy, from the way you act and look. I mean..." He thoughtfully placed his fingers on his chin and assumed the pose of a carnival man who runs the weight guessing game. "Okay, you've been in county jail for more than six months. Let's see, yes! Eating lots of garbage and candy has caused recent accumulation of serious fat!" He lightly touched my doughboy belly and uttered, "Tsk, tsk. No exercise to speak of and you seem to be...ah..." He held up his right forefinger and said, "Correct! That's it, distracted is the symptom! Of course that's from listening continually to a bunch of fools in County Jail." He shrugged a shoulder and clinically said, "That's a normal response."

I cracked a smile. "My man, you could work on any stage in any country."

With me playing along as his straight man, he felt safe continuing. He stepped close, squinted his eyes to look close at my skin, then shook his head sadly saying, "And you haven't seen the sun in all that time?" He raised his eyebrows mischievously. "Am I close?"

I stayed with him. In a serious tone I barked back, "I think you've been reading my mail! That's illegal man!"

He laughed. "Some are more obvious than others, and you're more so than most. Say Pops, how about some help carrying that stuff?"

"Yes, thanks."

"What unit are you in?"

"Unit? I don't know."

"Man, you *are* new. Okay, look, you've got a slip of paper

332

with the unit and cell you're assigned to on it."

"Oh, yeah, I got it right here." I pulled the slip from my pocket and with my hand shaking noticeably held it up to a light. "Says Unit 2-B."

"Terrific! You're progressing! Now you know where home is! I'm going that way. No problem. We'll be there in a few minutes. What's wrong with your hand? Sorry, but I can't help asking, are you nervous? Don't be. I mean this place is a piece of cake."

"Well, thanks, but no, not nervous exactly, just tired sort of, you know?"

"Hey, a couple of days and you'll be squared away."

"Thanks, thanks. I'll be okay." As we walked I watched other inmates just strolling casually around the compound. "Can everyone just walk around at night like this?"

"Sure, until 9:00 p.m. Not like County Jail, huh?"

I bent down, pulled a handful of fresh watered grass, then proceeded to fill my lungs. He snickered and said, "Hey, Dude, you ain't gonna eat that grass, are ya?"

I exhaled and laughed. "No, but it sure smells tasty! County Jail? Eight months. Eight stinking long, lousy months."

My new friend knew where I was coming from, and he grew more serious. "First time down?"

"Yeah, other than a couple of times for drinking and fighting when I got out of the service, but this is the first real time." The clean fresh air and scenery on the Sheridan Compound captivated me. "This place is beautiful, it looks like a park to me."

"You're right. Sheridan is considered a sweet place. It's new you know, I mean it's still prison, but not too bad. Not like State or a High Security joint. You've been through the worst physical part, now all you gotta do is learn how to do the time."

I glanced at him, and wondered what he really meant but said nothing. We walked.

Then he inquired, "If you don't mind my asking, how long you gonna be around?"

I couldn't imagine, relate or even utter the real answer. I only looked ahead. "A long time."

"Long time, huh? There's a lot of long time here."

We just strolled and said nothing for a while until he asked, "What's your name?"

We stopped walking for a moment when I turned to him. "Graham, Cano is my first name."

"Hmmm, that's Spanish, isn't it? You're not Mexican."

"Yeah, the name is Spanish, but no I'm not Mexican–it's a long story."

We continued walking, "Alright fair enough. Cano it is." He put my bag on his left shoulder and offered his hand. "They call me Bob 'The Little Ole Wine Maker' Bonds.

We shook hands. He laughed, glanced at my unruly mop of uncut gray hair and said, "Mr. Cano, you know what? If you ain't careful, you're gonna be white-haired before you get outta here."

We laughed. Bob made people laugh. I liked him.

Then he said, "Okay, here we are, this is 2-B. Just a second and I'll find someone to give you a hand. Do you need anything?"

"No thanks, I'm set. I've got it made."

We walked inside, and I found my cell. I smiled as I bounced and patted my mattress. Only someone who had been in my shoes knew how thrilled I was by the simple presence of a mattress and springs on a bunk bed.

Bobby said, "Okay, Mr. Cano, I've got to get outta here before I get written up for Out of Bounds. I live in Unit 3. Look Mr. Cano, I've got friends here. I mean I've talked to 'em already. They know you're here."

"Thanks, Bobby, I appreciate everything."

"It's nothing man, the worst is over. It'll take some time, but you'll settle in. See ya later."

Just as I finished putting my stuff away, a young inmate approached me. "Excuse me. Hi, you're Mr. Cano? I'm a friend of The Little Ole Wine Maker and, he told me to drop by. Hungry?"

He struck me as an eager young fella. "I'm Sidney from Portland."

"No, Sidney, I'm fine, but thanks anyway."

"Bob says you just came from County Jail, and he thought you might like a treat! How 'bout some hot-buttered popcorn–a whole bag–just out of the microwave!"

"My, my. Well Sidney, I can see you've definitely got my attention. Oh boy–hot-buttered popcorn? A whole bag?"

"Yep, sure enough!" Out from behind his back he produced a piping hot bag of delicious-smelling popcorn. All the while he smiled at my surprised reaction. "Mr. Cano, would you care for a soda?"

"Thanks, I never drink 'em."

"Oh really? You might like to know, we'll be having eggs and biscuits for breakfast and maybe bacon."

I was embarrassed by my right hand trembling badly, and I tried to still it by laying my hand flat on the bed. Sidney acted like he didn't see my difficulty in trying to open the bag. For a moment I thought he would offer to open it for me, but realized that would do more harm than good. I grabbed the bag, tore it open with my teeth and good hand, and grinned. Sidney made one more brief examination of the new senior addition on the compound, chuckled when he saw me diving into the popcorn, and said, "Okay! Enjoy, Mr. Cano. See ya at breakfast."

Through a mouth full of hot popcorn the muffled words came out, "Thanks, Sidney!"

He was a well-mannered young guy. I figured he was 22-23 years old and I wondered what his case was about.

I slept like a baby, didn't turn over, and was up early. I pulled on the orange coveralls issued to all new inmates, bummed a cup of coffee, and watched the morning news at 5:30 a.m. with six other interested souls. I felt like I had been released from prison rather than doing the first day of long time.

After another cup of donated coffee and 35 minutes of national news, the guy three chairs away who it seemed no one wanted to sit too close to said, "Okay, Pops, chow time!"

No one hesitated. Inmates walk faster to chow than at any other time. Many actually race to be ahead of the rest. It's a syndrome of sorts and frankly it appears like some primordial urge.

Interestingly enough, on that first morning I somehow found myself close to leading the charge for breakfast. I went eagerly through the line, got a complete breakfast of bacon, eggs, hash browns, and biscuits! Looking around the dining hall, I saw that all the tables were set up for four inmates. Terribly sophisticated.

For a moment I sat diligently still, just planning the all out attack on my breakfast. I suppose the orange coveralls and full tray gave me away as being brand new. I had already buttered and jellied my biscuits, set them aside, salt and peppered my eggs, and was about to dissect my eggs when a clean-cut middle-aged inmate approached my table.

"Good morning. Excuse me, may I join you?"

I noticed many other empty tables, but with plastic knife and fork held in a fashion that represented my weapons of choice, I looked up and thought, that's the first time in eight months that anyone has said, excuse me. Just as fast and actually overlapping that thought I placed my tools on my plate, smiled and said, "Sure, certainly. Have a seat."

He took a seat and instantly made what appeared an eccentric move. This fellow picked up one of his biscuits, and weighed the item in his hand. I didn't react. At that point he looked closely at the biscuit and took a nibble.

He savored the nibble for a few seconds, said, "Excuse me for a moment." He went back to the chow line where he engaged the cop on duty about something to do with the condition of our biscuits.

Now frankly at this point my interest in their debate lagged in view of the exquisite breakfast before me, which was completely full of sheer unadulterated goodness.

The biscuit connoisseur returned to the table, sat down, then

336

smiled the way one would while watching a kid with ice cream all over his face.

He cleared his throat and still smiling approvingly said, "Hungry? Tastes good, huh?"

Talking at this point was out of the question for me. Nodding had to suffice. I was busted with a mouthful of everything! Soon I worked it all around, took a large sip of coffee to wash most of it down, and said, "Yep! Whew! Sure does!" I winked and said, "Tastes great."

Then two other men joined us and the big burly one simply said, "Morning. How's the biscuits, Jeff?"

The Biscuit Connoisseur, a refined, self-assured sort of man who measured his words, stopped eating, put his utensils down and said to me, "Sorry, my name if Jeff. This is Doug and Tony."

We all nodded to confirm the introduction, "Hi, my name is Cano."

Another man approached the table, but when he saw it was full, he glanced at me, hesitated for a second and went on.

Doug was fiftyish, a big man, probably 275, with a receding hairline, thick glasses, a sour attitude, and I sensed a high IQ. Tony, a playfully passive little Mexican, appeared extremely bright and educated.

Jeff said, "They're heavy again, not enough flour." He laughed at the situation when he said, "I don't see why Clancy can't get it right. I just don't get it."

Tony just smiled at Jeff in an understanding manner and by so doing didn't give any notice to Jeff's comments, as if he had heard them before. He then turned to me and said, "Cano, C-A-N-O? Hmmm, that's a Mexican surname. Did you just drive up?"

"No, I didn't. You're the second one to ask me that, about driving here I mean." I looked at all three and said, "No way, they flew me all over: Chicago, El Reno, Salt Lake before we got to Portland. We took a bus here, that's the only driving I've done."

They looked at each other. "Do guys really drive up here and start doing time? Amazing!"

Tony cracked a slight smile and briefly caught the eyes of Doug and Jeff. By now I had gone back to my breakfast.

Jeff said in a sincere but curious manner, "Cano, excuse me, but how long have you been down?"

"I just got here last night."

"No, I mean all together."

"Oh, well, I was in County Jail for eight months."

Doug asked without looking up, "Eight months?"

"Yes, other than when I was a kid, then it was overnight."

Jeff had a serious and compassionate tone about him when he nodded and reflected with a certain understanding. "First time was eight months in County Jail? That's a long time, too long." He glanced at the others then back to me and said, in a way that was the first consoling words I'd heard, "Cano, we all know how you feel. Things will settle down fairly quick, the worst is over."

"Thanks, that's what I keep hearing."

I had started to think that Doug didn't care to ever make eye contact when he glanced up and in a blink back down to his breakfast asking, "Going to be with us long?"

Inmates have a natural curiosity about the length of a new man's sentence. The next unasked question is always, "What's your case about?"

The how long question penetrated and I resented having to answer, but I knew that a long time wouldn't do. I gave my answer quickly, afraid if I didn't respond promptly, I wouldn't at all.

The words felt like I was slicing the air when they came out: "Thirteen years, less good time."

They all grimaced at the same time. I felt their sympathy. Inmates have a way of indicating an emotion or reaction to such things as hearing the time one has given. Without undo emoting or audibly saying something like, "I'm sorry, man," they'll just squeeze their mouth or roll their eyes and grimace or grunt. That says it all.

I knew what they thought. I don't know what came over me. Maybe I was just tired of feeling down and of everything being so serious. Whatever, I saw a scene and decided to play it out.

I started to improvise. "Yeah, they hit me hard." I sighed to relieve the stress of confession and continued. "I've got this thing, this fixation like an all-consuming sexual obsession." I had their attention real good. I stroked my forehead in a pseudo-pensive style. "It finally got me busted."

Tony sat enthralled by my delivery, and Jeff and Doug were equally interested. It was little Tony who leaned over and half-whispered, "Well, what is it?"

I looked at each one, set my fork down, took a long sip of coffee and dead serious confessed. "I have this thing for streaking. I finally got caught with all my clothes off. Streaking in a Post Office!"

I had 'em. Each one of them! They looked at me dumbstruck. Completely blank.

"I know it's terrible, but I just love to do it, especially in a Post Office. I love to hear little old ladies scream! You know what I mean?" I looked for understanding in their eyes and only found incredulity.

During the next few seconds they all just sat back, slumped and searched each other for an answer they knew wasn't coming.

My timing was perfect. I held the moment for a second or so, then held up my hands in surrender, as if about to justify my sordid behavior, then at exactly the right time, I smiled and said, "Just kidding guys. Heh, heh, a little breakfast humor. Of course I'm not fooling about the thirteen years! By the way, it's for conspiracy and laundering money. I don't have the nerve to take my clothes off."

These guys burst out laughing and tried to keep from choking. Jeff stood up and covered his face with a paper napkin. Doug actually almost fell over backwards.

A cop came over, pleading, held out his hands and said, "Okay gentlemen, settle down, now what the hell is so funny this time of day?"

Doug started to answer, but started laughing again. Then he gathered himself and said, "We got hit, by a streaker in a Post…" and he started laughing.

Tony jumped in. "This fish just nailed all three of us with a story of streaking, and we bought it! Streaking in a US Post Office! Great! Can you imagine? And we bought it all!"

Now the cop bent over in laughter. Other inmates began laughing at these guys' laughing.

After a few minutes we had all settled down and Jeff asked, "Well, Cano, what was your main interest in the real world?" He smiled and said, "Now don't tell me it was hanging around the local Post Office."

"I got you guys good, huh? Heh, heh. You fellas probably never heard of my interest. Bottom line is, it all has to do with a special type of healing clay. Of course that was in the real world."

Doug and Tony glanced at Jeff as he said, "Really? Well I'll be." Jeff looked at Tony and Doug, then back to me saying, "Now that's interesting!"

I stood up ready to leave the table. "We'll have to talk about it sometime. It's been terribly important to me for several years. But of course now things are different with all this time. I shook hands with each of the men and said, "Hey, thanks a lot. Great to meet you guys, my first morning and all. Hey, I won't forget it. You fellas and my first biscuits in Federal Prison, seems both went down well."

Jeff stood up. "We enjoyed it too, really we did. If you need anything just let any of us know. We'll see you around Cano."

A day or so later Sidney approached me on the recreation yard. "Hey, Mr. Cano, you get around quick!"

"Hi, Sidney." Shaking hands I said, "How's that?"

"Those guys you had breakfast with on the first morning? Did you know 'em?"

"Why no, I just met 'em at breakfast. Nice guys. This man Jeff blew me away, though, I mean, I assumed he was joking for a second. Man, I never thought I'd see anyone carry on so about such good biscuits. I ate four of 'em. It was funny to me."

My young friend said, "Something was funny! Jeeze, the whole chow hall was laughing. Ha, even the cop! I was sitting two tables in back of you. I could tell you were enjoying the chow and Man! Mr. Cano, you said something that broke 'em all up. That was quite a time!"

"Well, Sidney, I pulled a little joke on 'em, that's what caused the whole thing."

Sidney was excited, "Yeah, well, you sure did. Plus, I mean those four guys have sat at that table for the last few years, and we all thought…"

"Four? There were only three."

"That's just it, Mr. Cano, that's part of the deal, you taking the table to start with! I mean you parked there with your orange jumpsuit on and all. Man, it was funny before it got funny! And then here comes Howard to take his normal place, ha! There you sat, not knowing what was going on. In his seat! I tell you this, some of us thought he was going to ask you to get up, and he would've except Jeff waved him off."

"He did? Jeff did that?"

"Sure he did. We all saw him. Doc knew you didn't know what time it was."

"What time was it?"

"Ah, Mr. Cano, that means you didn't know what was going on. It's just something we say."

"Oh, I got it, but who is Doc?"

"Jeff is Doc. You still don't know who he is, really?"

"Nope, sure don't. Doc? Jeff's a doctor? I mean is he a real doctor? What kind?"

"A doctor doctor! Mr. Cano, he's Dr. Jeffrey McDonald!"

"Hmmm, sorry Sidney, but it doesn't ring a bell. McDonald?"

"Mr. Cano, he's famous! Surely you've heard of him. He's doing three life terms. They say he killed his wife and two daughters. He's like a movie star, you know, a celebrity after being on TV and all."

"Wait a minute Sidney! McDonald. The Captain in the Green Berets?"

"Yes, that's what I'm saying, that's him!"

"Really? I saw the TV story, *Fatal Something*, wasn't it?"

"You got it Mr. Cano. Tell me, do you think he did it? You know, killed 'em all?"

"Aw, Sidney, I don't know about all that. I mean who knows? Frankly I wasn't really into that story to begin with, but as I remember, this writer of the book, what's his name, anyway he turned rat and jerked the Doctor around real good. It seems he slanted the story badly against Doctor McDonald."

"Yeah, that's what a recent article said, too. My mom told me that."

"Since you mention it, seems like I recall reading last year that the lawyers for Jeff have a new book coming out that creates one hell of a compelling case for his defense."

Sidney said, "Right, they do! I believe it's called *Fatal Justice* or something like that. We all like him. He's a ball playing fool, and always helping someone, you know with medical stuff. In fact he actually saved the life of an inmate once."

"Well I'll be damned! The Biscuit Connoisseur is Dr. McDonald, small world. Sidney, who're the other two, who's the big guy?"

Sidney loved giving the hot scoop about what I didn't know. "Okay, Mr. Cano, they call him the Prof. I don't really know him, he seems to be pissed about something all the time. I understand he was a real professor in Washington somewhere. I understand that his girlfriend ratted him out to the Feds, and they caught him inside his warehouse full of grass plants. He had everything all rigged up electronically. Mr. Cano, he even canned his grass. Can you

342

imagine? He put it up in tin cans. It was all real slick I guess." He laughed. "Except he forgot they were watching his electric bills besides listening to his young girlfriend. He thinks he's better than most of us. I don't like him, and not many do for that matter."

"What about the Mexican guy? He seems friendly enough."

"Oh, he is. Always having fun, messing around. I understand he and Doc became friends when they were in Bastrop, Texas together, and wound up here. I knew he got a lot of time for flying drugs in. He's supposed to have been real bad at one time, but now he's a neat guy, a real good artist too."

"You know a lot Sidney. How old are you?"

"I'm 21, at least I'll be 21 in a month and a half."

He seemed so young, because he was so young. I felt ancient yet complimented when he frowned, squinted and asked, "Mr. Cano, are you going to call me Sidney?"

"Not if you don't want me to. "

"Oh, no, it's okay. It's just that here nobody calls me anything but Sid. My mom always calls me Sidney. It's okay if you do too. It's all right."

"What does your dad call you?"

"He used to call me Sidney too, but he hasn't been around since I was in the 7th grade. He married another lady and moved down South to California. I have a step-dad now, a long-haul trucker. He calls me Sid, but it's fine with me, if you call me Sidney."

"Well, all right! Sidney it is!"

He stuck out his fist, and at that moment with Sidney, I "hit the hammer." We sealed our friendship.

Chapter 44

What Might Have Been

Make the most of your regrets—
to regret deeply is to live afresh.

Henry David Thoreau

Those first eight months in county did far more psychological damage than I realized at the time. The absolute trauma of losing my freedom, along with everything I had created, then devastated by the sheer grief of Mom's passing, and our dreams smashed, resulted in a bitter futility. Coping with these life-altering circumstances within the demeaning confines of an old, over-crowded, mid-western jail, forced me to withdraw and seek an uninvolved safe haven. But I was vulnerable, couldn't hide my nature, and was exposed as being who I am.

My inherent optimism, and high regard and respect for my fellows began to crumble like a cracked china teacup, slowly draining my energy. In that stifling setting, many of the inmates confused simple kindness and decency with weakness. Their primitive and barbaric interpretation began to fester and grow unchecked, way out of balance. I was out of control.

The experience came to represent a morbid example of the rampant dreck in our species' character.

Deplorable human behavior aside, much of the first few weeks

344

in federal prison seemed an elaborate sort of wonderful fantasy. No doubt conceived through a severe form of denial, nonetheless, I unconsciously concocted an emotional escape hatch that to some degree allowed me to compare my new Federal Prison adventure with the drama of being sentenced to some secluded foreign legion outpost.

I mean, after all, in my new utopian outpost I could sleep! Inmates wore clean uniforms, ate nourishing food, and enjoyed sufficient housing. Everyone had a job, adequate recreation, and library access. No one asked too many questions, and most notably, most inmates offered proper respect when the same was received. No question about it, this outpost was far removed from and a vast improvement over the insanity and cages of county jail!

Ah, yes! But the presence of cold reality has a subtle manner of crashing uninvited through even the most exotic of one's dream.

Predictably, the newness of Federal Prison began to wear thin, biscuits and all! This was no fabled silver screen outpost. I was down, pure and simple. I woke up early one rainy Oregon morning, and realized that although this wasn't county jail, Federal Prison was serious business. When I emotionally surfaced for air, I focused on their icy cold razor wire and doing long time, rather than on my private diversion.

And then one day over the institution's sound system, I heard my name called. "Graham - 97079-012. Come to the chaplain's office."

I knew this couldn't be good. When I got there, he told me my brother was dead. My little brother, Dr. Frank, had been killed in a plane crash. I was through. I had thrown away a promising acting career, lost my dream of a Therapeutic Clay Research Center/Healing community, my mother, and now my only living brother was gone. I was alone, the last surviving member of W.L. and Eva Graham's family of six.

Restless nights became meandering weeks. I felt entombed with no viable history, no functional future, and no interest in today.

Emotionally exhausted, I continued to shuffle forlornly around the graveled running track, hating the company of others. I hated going in circles. I always walked alone straight out and straight back. Every unconscious lap was like an added thread for the cocoon of my dangerous emotional state. Aimlessly I walked, drowning in the nostalgic morass that begins with "The saddest words of tongue or pen" and ends with the heartbreak of "what might have been."

Chapter 45

Hooked-Up

Men Talk about Bible miracles because there is no miracle in their lives. Cease to gnaw that crust. There is ripe fruit over your head.

Henry David Thoreau

I kept to myself for several weeks. I ate alone, walked alone, worked alone, and grieved. I wasn't the first, I wouldn't be the last, but nonetheless the inmates understood and treated me with respect as I struggled for my emotional breath.

As soon as I began serving my sentence, Ruthie Badame and Silvia Burton sent cheerful and thoughtful letters, which I took to the recreation yard. I walked the track reading them, wept where no one would notice, and learned that pain creates pain as fire feeds on fire. I could not or would not put the hurt away.

I don't know what I'd have done without Ruthie during that black period of my life. Her letters were full of encouragement and news from Tecopa Hot Springs. She always included a full page of jokes, cartoons clipped from the paper, and particularly interesting articles as well. She remained very in tune to the local gossip, and kept me informed about the people we knew, and who asked about me.

She kept telling me, "I won't let them forget you, Cano. Not ever."

I couldn't stop the tears when I read her letters. No matter my difficulties, Ruthie believed in me and constantly reaffirmed that God heard her prayers and was watching out for both of us. I called her on the phone as well, and she helped me get through days when nothing else seemed to work.

Ultimately, however, she admitted in the midst of one of her long letters, that she wasn't feeling well. I could only imagine what that meant for the time being. She continued writing to me every two weeks, and then one day, she simply told me that she had lung cancer. She had begun what would become a two-year battle for her life. Her letters didn't slow up, though, and from the first day that we met, to the last, she remained a true and loyal friend.

After she checked into the hospital for chemotherapy, we remained in communication. As she slipped away, she showed tremendous courage and held firmly to her faith in God. And, in that condition, physically weakened and suffering from the various side effects of the radiation therapy, Ruthie achieved an important victory for clay therapy.

She hated chemo, and it drove me mad to imagine her ordeal. I'd taken an intense interest in researching clay application in cancer patients. I found it helped not only stress relief, but helped stop post-treatment infections, improve hygiene, and especially detoxify the system from the side effects of chemo. In Ruthie's case, it helped her mouth infections.

One night, I called her from Sheridan Federal Prison to talk with her. She was going through hell and complained about the sores in her mouth.

I remember shouting, "For God's sake, can't they give you something to stop a simple sore in your mouth?"

"Cano, the antibiotics don't help."

"Ruthie, our clay will take care of any infections in your mouth. How are your gums?"

"Bad, Cano, very bad."

I couldn't understand it. I felt confused, angry, and helpless. I pulled myself together long enough to make some calls, and within a few hours, Ruthie had our therapeutic clay in her mouth.

One of the most exciting days of my life came the very next time I called back, and heard my precious friend say, "It's working. Cano, I wish you were here. The nurses and doctors can't believe it. Our Mexican orderly calls it a miracle, a gift from God! Our clay is working! Cano, are you still thinking about writing a book about Tecopa Hot Springs and the clay?"

"Yes, dear, I sure am. Someday."

"Good, don't forget to mention how well it works for chemo patients."

"I'll remember, sweetheart. I'll remember. Get some rest."

Ruthie and I spoke with each other on the phone just eighteen hours before she passed away. She finally said she was ready to go. We had a bad connection, though, and she kept yelling, "Keep chipping away, Cano. Don't quit! I love you. I love you."

"I love you too, Ruthie. Always."

The line went dead. Our time was up.

A fellow inmate said, "Hey, man, what's wrong? Are you okay?"

I broke down and sobbed. I was losing my precious friend, and I prayed to the Power that one day I could tell her story.

After Ruthie's death, I escaped to the library for hours at a time into the world of old *National Geographic* magazines only to come around actually surprised by being surrounded with federal inmates. I wasn't interested in newspapers. I didn't want or care to know about the real world and what was happening, because I was no longer a part of the community.

I came to believe the spirit of my very being was drifting unattached, withdrawing, and shriveling away. I couldn't admit to myself or anyone else, how frightened and despondent I was becoming.

Over the next few years, Sylvia Burton also passed away. She was loved in her community as a solid citizen, a beautiful woman, and a fine artist. I love her for just being Sylvia, my second mom.

While serving my time in prison, Art and Luella Babbitt, Beulah Rosenberg, Joyce Lassos, and Curt Hibdon also died. Oh, how I miss them! How fortunate I was to have known and loved them.

As became my daily pattern, I was on the track kicking little rocks and strolling in four hundred forty-yard circles. A threatening rainstorm had blown in from the Oregon coast, and a few isolated drops caused the other inmates to scurry for cover leaving me thankfully alone. What a relief to be alone. I thoroughly welcomed the few warm marble-sized sprinkles because they were a guarantee of solitude. The rare opportunity of being alone in prison is similar to enjoying a dark night inside the razor wire. Neither ever happens.

I closed my eyes and raised my face to the low hanging clouds as the big plush drops splattered. I took the splashes personally as if they were aimed just for me. The sun peeked out in spots as the big sprinkles turned into a fast moving, but gentle shower.

I turned up my collar, rechecked the track to make sure I was still alone, looked skyward again, and although somewhat surprised and self-conscious realized I was about to do something I had never actually done before.

Suddenly I yelled out loud. "Honey, I need to talk! Come in!"

For the past several months I had practiced this ritual of visualizing and having a conversation of sorts with Mom, but usually those moments were when I was about to fall asleep, and filled with my grief rather than a real two-way conversation. Grieving precludes listening.

Amazingly, as if in some computer generated science fiction scene, mother came in.

At first, the image came like witnessing a rainbow where one can see the rainbow, but see through it also. Slowly everything in the picture began to clear up. The apparition fascinated me, and I watched it all on a huge television-like screen levitating just inches above the gravel and not more than a few yards in front of me. I clearly saw Mom talking to friends at a dining table, but as if in a nonsensical dream I imagined she couldn't see or hear me.

I waited a moment, looked briefly around the recreation yard, and a bit quieter, anxiously repeated, "Honey, can you hear me? Come in!"

In a matter of seconds she waved like always and smiled at me. She then leaned toward her friends and said, "Excuse me please, my son Cano is calling. I don't want him to break off. It's his first time." She got up, walked briskly over to a big wooden chair sitting outside the dining area, and sat down facing me.

Mother appeared surprisingly at ease as if this were normal. Then a stagehand attached a small microphone on her blouse. I knew she must be excited but she was still perfectly at ease. In a tone like an old hand at this business Mom inquired, "Is this working? I mean are we on?" Mother was a little impatient and pointedly asked, "Sir, can my son hear me?"

A voice off camera said, "Yes, Mrs. Graham, go ahead."

With that signal she smiled, waved vigorously, and sang out a bright, "Helloooo!"

She seemed loud. I glanced around the yard, moved just my hand and fingers, and surprised myself by saying rather meekly, "Hi, Honey. I hear you just fine. In fact, you can even have them turn the sound down." I wondered if anyone else could hear her. "And Honey, I see you clear as day."

I wondered, what do you say to your mother in this situation?

I looked at that expressive face and said, "Mom you look great! I mean the last time I saw you, well you were so tired."

Mom laughed at my description. "That's a nice way of saying that I looked like death warmed over." She chuckled again. "Yes, dear, I can imagine how I looked. I was tired, but mainly I was mad because they wouldn't fix my hair before you came." She shrugged a shoulder. "Anyway, it's not important now. That's all history."

"History or not that was the toughest day of my life!"

"Oh Honey, I knew it was difficult for you while it was

351

happening but there was nothing I could do. I've learned since that we can't deny those we love the grieving process. It's against the law here no matter how much we'd like to have our loved ones accept it easier. The real problem though, from what I see, is that you still haven't accepted the whole thing. I swear, you hold onto things, good or bad, longer than any of the boys. You always did." She grew more serious. "Harry you're wasting time, and time is so important. I'm so glad you're tuning in! We need to talk."

"Honey, you called me Harry. You haven't called me Harry in twenty years!"

"I did, didn't I? I was thinking of you when you were a little boy." She smiled, again having fun with the moment. "Just slipped out I guess." Then she squirmed in her chair. "Honey, isn't this fun!"

"Yes, sweetheart, it's a lot of fun, but you know it's way different than I imagined. I mean, simply talking this way and all, and being able to see you, it's like you're real."

She shot back, "Thinking is real, isn't it?"

"Yeah I guess so. Sure it is."

"Well, then I'm real!" She giggled again. "I got you thinking–huh?" She reached to her right side and plugged a cord into a little cedar box.

I was curious, "What's that for, the box??"

She smiled and said, as if patting herself on the back, "Your momma has a direct line to the power!" She then leaned towards me and whispered privately, "It seems to go on a point system of some kind. Ha! Anyway, I'm in and if I'm in the loop, then you're in also!" Mom was having a delightful time when she said, "If you get it, you got it! And we got it!!"

Now she had me going. "Mom that's neat! You're saying that you can be like my go-between with the main power source? And make sure I get through with a clear solid, connection?"

"Yep!" She was milking this for all it was worth. "I can do that and more!"

Somehow our relationship was different. She was doing for me rather than me for her. I realized I couldn't do for her except in the sense of what I could do for myself.

"Mom this is all so unbelievable! I mean, you seem to know what I've been through. I tell you it's been a..."

She broke in which wasn't like her. "You've been resisting beyond normal, that's what you've been doing, Cano. Dear, it's time to snap out of it. Lord knows, excuse the pun, but you've been hard at work for some time freely giving your energy and power away to the wrong places. Recently, I've learned the way it always works, and well I must say, if that's your choice, so be it. I mean, no one can stop you, but I hate to see and know you're suffering so."

I checked the track again to make sure no one was near. "So you know what my biz was all about out there, and where I am now?"

"Oh, I knew something was up, I mean you weren't acting, and lots of money was coming in, but I want you to know something, I had great fun counting the five dollar bills!" She laughed. It was wonderful to hear her laugh.

Mother raised her hand to indicate an interruption was coming when into the scene came a darling little black girl, eight or nine years old wearing a bright yellow spring dress with matching ribbons in her hair. She was bringing mother a tray with coffee and cream. The little girl carefully set the silver tray by the cedar box on the small table beside mother.

Mother smiled at the bashful girl and said, "Thank you, Ginger."

Ginger curtsied ever so properly, and then self-consciously smiled at me, and skipped off camera.

"I told Ginger all about how I knew you'd love her. She's been anxious for you to hook-up. Isn't she precious?"

"She certainly is! But honey is this all in my mind? Are you really there? Is Ginger really there too?"

"I understand your question, Honey. You just don't entirely get it yet."

"The problem is that I just don't..."

Again, unlike her usual self, mom said, "What you don't get yet is the simple fact that if I'm in your mind then I'm real, or I couldn't come in. What part of that don't you understand?"

I grinned. "Hey, Gal, don't get testy."

She smiled in her loving fashion. "Honey, just trust what I'm saying, plus what you've always believed in. Hook-up often with your momma and you'll see the light." She said this playfully while shaking a finger at me.

I took a deep breath, exhaled, and said, "Okay, Honey, I'm willing."

"Oh, I'm so happy! Now about this matter of your Biz and how I felt about it? I've thought about this issue, and frankly when I saw you putting your clay on people, what it meant to them and you, well I wasn't the only one who could see that you were creating something of worth. At first when I saw all the money I was concerned with your motivation, but soon enough I saw what you were doing. I knew you were still the same person as the little boy trying to save the frog and feeling bad about the mouse drowning so I decided to support you no matter what. That was my choice!

"Nothing is either all good or all bad, there's a trade off. Certain principals are why laws change, and you were doing more good than bad. Anyway that's the way I feel. That's not to say it wasn't against the law of the land, and for that you got a thirteen-year sentence."

I looked around the yard. "Mom, this is too much. Am I hallucinating? At first I kinda assumed all this was coming from me, but I'm not so sure."

"Oh, you're in charge of your end. I mean you have to ask for me to come in, but once cleared I take over from here." She motioned to include all the others in the room. "We never go where we're not invited, or until the one who is inquiring is ready to receive. The sad part is that many here who can give the most are never even asked. It's just terrible not to be asked."

"I can understand that feeling, but what if someone asks, but isn't really ready to listen?"

"In that case, that someone's dumpster isn't completely empty and he isn't yet ready or willing to trust the process. Like I said, we aren't allowed to come until one is truly ready. No one is out of place. It's sad to see, but we hear about it happening all the time."

This explanation bothered me "Damn! What do you mean by ready? Ready for what?"

"Ready simply means being ready to trust your law."

"Aw, come on, Mom. What law?"

"Now, Honey, don't worry. The law means whatever spiritual belief one has. For instance you believe in what is called Universal Law. That's clear enough, and fine and dandy. But we've got all sorts of different beliefs here. Some a bit strange, but it doesn't matter a hoot which is your choice. What matters is the extent of your trust in what you believe. I might add that it seems to us that enough pain will usually create a willingness to trust in something."

I turned around on the track, kicked some gravel, and shook my head cussing at the world in general. "This is the damnedest thing I've ever seen."

Mom tried to settle me down. "I don't know why this surprises you so. We've talked about it before. In fact, you were the first one to tell me the exact same thing." In a more subdued tone she said, "Honey, it's just that now it's not theory or conversation, it's what we call crunch time."

I blurted out, "Crunch time? When did you start using a term like crunch time?"

Mom was truly kind of sassy when she smiled and said, "Just now because it fits. Ha! Seriously dear, most are not close to being ready, but in your case the misery index plus the fact that you've asked for divine intervention says you've had enough, are ready, and willing." She raised both hands above her head and yelled. "Whoopee! Here I am. Here we are! By the way, Mister, you look terrible, I mean like a sixty year old man that's been…"

"Mom! I am a sixty-year-old man!"

"I know, but you don't have to look like a wreck."

She was playing with me, shaking her head in false disgust, but with a serious undertone. "How long has it been since you did any exercise or ran for a half-hour?"

"I've been in county jail, lady! It's been awhile. I just…"

"And candy! I can't believe your sweet tooth. When did you get hooked on Snickers?"

"Aw, I just kinda…" I felt she was enjoying this banter.

"And sleeping during the day when you haven't done any work to be the least bit tired from. I don't know what's gotten into you."

"Okay. Okay! I got it. Come on Honey, give me a break. I'm just not over losing everything and you being gone. I can't seem to get going."

She motioned to include the dining room and said, "We all understand. Yours is a normal reaction, but you're overdoing it! I'm glad you asked me in, because in some of the strongest people this problem can become habitual."

"I just can't seem to…"

She wouldn't let me finish. "Please, Cano, listen to me. I love you so. More than my life. Don't you know I've been watching? I just couldn't come in, Dear. Lately you've been close a few times, but you can't seem to let go completely and trust the Power that you've always believed in. I know you've never believed anything else, but in this adversity if you don't rededicate, reaffirm and recommit 100% every day to what you instinctively believe, then the price will be continued unresolved pain. This adversity is part of the process for you. You have a long way to go in your journey. Continue to hold the truth of the law in its proper place as a guide, but step away trusting, raise the bar, and get in action. Remember, sweetheart like you once told me, 'Trust is the great adventure.' Don't you remember?"

"Yeah, I remember, but now…"

"Honey, you've already honestly made the first and most critical step."

"Wait a minute. I have? What was it?"

She stood up, adjusted the cushion in her chair, sat back down and said, "Do you remember the night when you were half asleep and whispered, 'God help me!' Then for a few moments you were thinking of me and asking for divine intervention and inspiration? Remember?"

"Yeah, I recall it was late one night. You know, Mom it was like I'd finally surrendered. I had nothing left. I was powerless."

Mom almost came out of her chair, "Exactly! You hooked-up in that second. I don't know if you're aware or not, but your genuine, heart-felt supplication for God to help you turned the tide."

"That did it? Hell, I would've asked a lot sooner if I'd known it was that easy."

"Come on now, you can't cut any corners to get there. That's why you're where you are. One has to really be there, and you had genuinely emptied your dumpster of despair, and were finally willing to reload with fresh fuel. It took you long enough."

"Mom, you're a straight up trip." I looked around the yard and mumbled, "This is something else." Then with my hands on my hips in a light hearted but defensive posture, I asked, "Mom, do you mean I get another shot?"

She laughed. "Honey, you've got many shots left!"

"I do? Well I'll be darned. Hey! Do I really look bad?"

She tightened her lips. "You look like an out of shape, fat, sixty-year-old man, next case."

"Next case? Whoa there! You seem a bit extreme."

"Extreme or not, you look too fat." Now she pushed the dig,

saying with great emphasis, "And extremely soft."

"Mom!"

"You asked! Don't ask if you can't stand to know the answer!"

"Hey, lady, don't they practice diplomacy or tact up there?"

She gestured with her forefinger, smiled "gotcha" style, and said, "In the first place I'm not up there, and second, yes! We try to be tactful but we don't patronize. It's counter productive."

"My, my, it's that cut and dried?"

"Yes, but there's something else we need to discuss. It has to do with getting away from just talk, talk, think, think. It has to do with action."

"Action? What kind of action?"

"You'll have new direction and guidance, and you need it because you've been thinking too much without enough action."

"Mom, what are you talking about?"

"Okay, Dear, let me ask you a simple question. Let's assume you were going to be released in six months and were offered the lead role in a play on Broadway? What's the first thing you'd do tomorrow?"

"Aw, come on, Mom, you know what I'd do. Hell, I'd start preparing tonight and continue till we opened! Hey, just a moment, what are you saying? Do you know something I should know? Have you got agents there, too?"

"No, Cano, we don't have agents! But I can remind you of something real that you seem to have forgotten. Agents? How silly!"

"Well, I didn't know. You seem to have a bag full of tricks."

"What I'm talking about is no trick, no dream and no joke. Honey, it's time for you to seriously start digging your trenches where you are. Start preparing for the flood of prosperity if you truly trust the power!"

"Mom, I told you that story of digging our trenches, and preparing for the flood, but Hell, I'm in prison! What can I do about anything? I'll end up doing ten or eleven years on a thirteen-year sentence. That's what's in front of me! Dammit!"

Mother put both hands up and said, "Whoa, Honey, you can't what? You've got a life in front of you, inside the fence or not, a life--a good productive life. You're one of the lucky ones. You'll see that you have a life! Honey, think about the truth of what I'm saying. Life means choices, and choices for you means creating! Please don't tell the Power you've got nothing to give, that you choose nothing. She'll answer you! Please don't think or say that. It frightens me because it's so dangerous."

She started to quietly cry which made me feel like a real scrooge. I didn't know what to do.

A voice from off camera said, "Go ahead, child take it to her."

Ginger came onto the scene carrying a handkerchief and gave it to her. Ginger was pouting and her lower lip was quivering. She cast me an accusing look.

Mother took the handkerchief, gave Ginger a hug, and told her she was all right.

After Ginger left, mother dabbed her eyes and said, "Oh, Honey, this is so important, you must understand something. The Power never discriminates and is very impersonal. Please believe and trust this: the Power, the Light, the Force, God the Creator, whatever name you wish, whatever! And no matter who or where, the law of this universe will seldom give you exactly what you might think you want, but will always give you what you choose. When you choose, you trust. And when trust is there you expect it! And only then do you receive what you've chosen! Done deal!"

"Done Deal? When did you start saying done deal? Whew! I mean Mom, I've never heard you talk this way before."

"It's just that I've never been good at speaking my feelings, but now that I'm here, and in the loop of being hooked-up well, it's all different. Don't you like what I'm saying? We've discussed most of the very same thing before, many times in fact."

"I can't make sense of all this. I was prepared to go through this whole thing ..."

She interrupted me again. "Dear, excuse me, but what's hard to accept is that your dumpster is finally empty. Kaput! It's over! You've drained it of most all the hurt. Oh, some of the memories will hang around, but their influence will be harmless when you're in action."

I just couldn't believe how she was going on. Kaput? She never said kaput in her life. Where'd that come from? I mean who is she hanging around? "So, with that said, young man, you're faced with realizing the divine intervention and inspiration you asked for is happening here and now! Choices are on the menu, sir. Thank you."

I couldn't slow her up. "Mom, about my clay..."

She wouldn't let me talk. "You must prepare for emotional, physical and creative prosperity."

"But, Mom what about..."

"Dear, your plan isn't working too good! Right?"

I threw my arms out to include the entire compound and said, "Hey, gal! You got that right. I mean, look around."

"Alright, the point is, why would you ask for divine intervention and inspiration if you didn't believe that by so doing, the laws would manifest a positive life beyond your present scope?"

"Well, I..."

"Please dear, don't make the fatal mistake of putting the cart ahead of the horse by trying to direct the Power."

"Mother, I'm simply trying to figure how to..."

"Cano, stop! Quit thinking! First, accept the Power's gift of life itself and in so doing respect the intrinsic universal laws or truths that apply to everyone whether we like it or not! These inherent universal truths represent the essence, the substance between cause and effect that all the great prophets and thinkers have referred to for the past 2000 years! And longer! We take classes on this subject!"

She left me dumbfounded. She had said more in these few minutes than all of her life together concerning such matters.

She leaned forward in her chair. "Son, I know you believe and fully appreciate what we've discussed, but believing alone and truly appreciating these truths isn't enough. Belief and appreciation without action is an exercise in escapism."

Ginger came into the scene again with a glass of water for mom and carrying a small sign. After setting the water down she cupped her hand to her chest and waved to me. Ginger then turned the sign around that read:

> Hi, Cano, I'm sorry I frowned at you.
> I'm happy you're hooked-up
> Ginger

I waved back. "Thanks, Ginger, that's sweet of you."

She skipped off camera again as I turned to mother and said, "Now, Honey, don't interrupt me please! You know how important the clay was to me. Now that I'm here, I can't really do anything."

She did it again! "Honey, do you realize you just said 'was' to me and then 'I can't?' Be careful with your thoughts. Remember the Power is very impersonal. Those thoughts are registered and they're powerful. Be careful." She glanced around and included her friends. "We've discussed you and the clay, what it *is*, not *was*, to you, and what you *can*, not *can't*, do now. It's interesting for everyone to realize the extent of what clay therapy could mean to so many, but what no one comprehends is why you feel so thwarted to continue the effort where you are."

"Why? Mom, I'm in Federal Prison."

"Honey, didn't you say that Ralph Waldo Emerson once said, 'You must demonstrate where you are.' Didn't he say that?"

"Ah, yes, yes he did." I thought, among a whole lot of other things I don't care to confront.

She continued. "Right! And I know your body is in prison, but your mind and heart are free. The court says you broke the law and

361

you did. Granted the court ruled that you do thirteen years in prison, but the court didn't say *how* you do your time, or what you can or can't create. Your prison time is the court's business, how or what you create while here is your business."

"But, Honey, I don't have my clay here."

"Cano, you don't need the clay to actually be there to gather information, and tell your clay story. After all, your subject of Clay Therapy and all of your experience didn't go to prison. You did!"

"But how?"

"You've told me you have a lot of important unanswered questions about where, how, when and why clay therapy would be extremely useful, especially to those who can't afford doctors or medicine. Ginger is one of those."

"Really? What happened?"

"A simple infection turned to blood poisoning. It need not have happened! Her mom couldn't afford medicine and before she realized how serious it was, Ginger was gone. It's not rare, happens all the time."

"What a shame! A life taken so early."

"Dear, think about all the information in your head not in any books, and all the experiences you used to tell me about. Those would be important for lots of people to hear. You told me more than once about the healing power of clay."

At that moment, the institution's loudspeaker blared. "Attention in the Institution. Yard Recall! Yard Recall!" Then in the same cold robotic tone, "All inmates return to their housing units for count time. Count time!"

The noise startled me for a second, then the huge bubble burst and pulled me back into the present. I looked for mom but she was gone. There was no screen, no nothing. It was as if I had been jarred awake from a dream that was life-like, the kind one remembers.

I had not even noticed the sunny, cloudless sky until this moment. I took in a deep breath of sweet air and noticed the lightness of my spirit. My visit with Mom had certainly done me good. For the past year when I groomed myself, I usually felt emotionally the same way I appeared outwardly. The hooked-up episode instantly messed with that equation. When I paused by a window on the gym, happily heading for my unit, I was astounded by the illusion of seeing another man in my reflection. I no longer felt the same as the person coming back at me. For the first time since my incarceration, I lightly stepped on the inmates' scales inside the gym, and realized I had gained thirty pounds.

I weighed 225 pounds. I stepped off to view myself in a full-length mirror only to see the truth of what I had become, and deeper, I saw me, the cause of it all.

I stood there blankly looking at myself, turned from side to side, and repeated over and over and over Emerson's profound words: "As within so without. As within so without."

Doc McDonald had been working out on the weights. As he was leaving the gym he passed me and said, "Hey, Cano, I need to talk with you! How you been doing?" Referring to me on the scales he said, "Checking things out?"

I felt a bit silly standing in front of the mirror so long. I turned to him and said, "Yeah, Doc, I'm appraising the damage."

He laughed. "Ah! It could be worse."

"Hmmmm."

Doc said, "Seriously, you're ahead of the game already."

I turned away from the mirror to face him. "Oh? How?"

"You're diagnosing the problem!" He laughed as he toweled off.

I turned back to the mirror. "Well, there's a lot to operate on."

"How've you been? What's new?"

"Not much, Jeff, pretty quiet for me. I've just been taking a little walk. I do a lot of that."

Jeff smiled as if he knew or had seen something, but didn't react further.

"Doc, you mentioned us talking about the clay."

"Oh, yes. This will surprise you. I'd like to walk a few laps and discuss clay therapy with you."

His interest pleased me. "Great, anytime. Be glad to."

"Thanks. My girlfriend is into holistic medicine, has been for some time. Anyway I told her about your interest in Clay Therapy. One thing led to another and it turns out her daughter in Las Vegas has been to your place in Tecopa Hot Springs. She had a skin problem that medicine wouldn't touch. She said a lady named Joyce was in charge at the time and showed her how to clear it up."

"Well, get outta here!" I stepped away from the man in the mirror. "Jeff, you're kidding!"

"No! Really surprised me too. Cano, I'd like to know more. My girlfriend would like to sell it maybe."

"Doc, I'd be glad to tell you what I know. It's fascinating and definitely interesting for anyone, but with your medical training, well, you may be quite surprised. I've already put the subject out of my mind, but I'll put some notes together and we'll talk."

We shook hands and he said, "Good, good, we'll do it. Okay, thanks, see you at chow."

"All right, we're on. See you then."

Jeff left me still considering the two figures. The one in my mind and the one in the mirror. One of us was about to depart this world, and I thought, "It ain't gonna be me."

Once a man fully realizes that he can mold only the day he has, or if other days, only through it, he will begin both to take things easily and to do them well, and these two have a closer connection than most people seem to imagine.

Joseph Farrell, Irish clergyman

Chapter 46

A Victory Lap

Apparent failure may hold in its rough shell the gems of a success that will blossom in time, and bear fruit throughout eternity.

Frances Ellen Watkins Harper

I soon developed an early morning routine, my ritualistic rock and blessing for the next two years in Sheridan Federal Prison. When the unit doors opened for chow at 6:00 a.m., I went directly to the pea-graveled quarter mile running track. I set the rhythm for this private time by easily shuffling along, and whispering the classic lines of a longtime favorite poem, Benjamin Disraeli's inspiring words:

Salutation to the Dawn

Look to this day for it is life
The very life of your life.
In its brief course runs all of the
Verities and realities of your existence.
The bliss of growth
The glory of action
The splendor of beauty.
For yesterday is but a dream

Tomorrow is only a vision.
But today well lived,
Makes every yesterday a dream of happiness
And every tomorrow a vision of hope.
Look well therefore to this day
And such is the salutation to the new dawn.

It seemed like I could always hear a rooster crowing by the time I finished the poem and had progressed to a full jog. About this time, Mom came in for a brief two or three minute chitchat about miscellaneous events before hooking me up. After we signed off I examined the specifics of my day, put everything in order, finished my run, and eagerly headed for breakfast, my favorite meal of the day.

With my breakfast tray all squared away, I looked for a spot to land when I noticed Jeff waving for me to join him and Doug.

I set my tray down. "Thanks. Morning, gentlemen."

They both replied, "Morning, Cano."

"All right, the first thing I need to know is how's the biscuits?"

Jeff grinned as if it wasn't a real issue. "They're learning." He added, "It just takes time."

Doug cracked a half smile. Jeff immediately got to business. "Cano, I'm pleased to say my girlfriend got your clay last week, but told me something which I frankly question." He saw Tony in the chow line and with one finger waving, let him know we had a seat for him. "We need your input."

I started to butter my biscuits. "Okay, Doc, fire away."

"You said it worked well on various skin problems. I understand the application fine, but have you ever known the clay to be used as a primary treatment for pain such as arthritis?"

I glanced at Jeff, then at Doug, and back to Jeff. "Have I ever used my clay to treat arthritis?" I broke out into a huge grin. "Are you serious?"

Jeff said, "Oh yes, there's a serious debate in progress here. I mean my girlfriend has an elderly neighbor with arthritic fingers, and she actually found relief with the clay. I told her the reaction was possibly a placebo effect. The question I have is what do you think about such a claim? I mean we're talking arthritis!"

"So? Jeff, arthritics were some of the first and most devoted disciples of what we were doing with our clay. I mean seriously! You can take it to the bank. Clay is very effective, plus fast acting, on many types of arthritis, and joint pain in general for that matter, no question about it! That sort of topical application is fundamental with clay therapy."

Bordering on sarcasm, Doug quietly knifed in "Disciple? Who coined that phrase?" Doug had a rude habit of sometimes eating and watching his food rather than looking at the person he was speaking to.

I let his attitude slide. "Doug, it was actually my mom."

He turned to Jeff, "You know I like that. Disciple? Hmmm. Your mom? Well that's neat."

Jeff was a bit preoccupied, and his habit of unconsciously brushing the spot on his temple surfaced when he said, "So this isn't new to you at all?"

"Hardly! Real common use in fact." I grinned. "But I'm always pleased to hear of happy customers spreading the word. She'll find many other uses as well. Everything in the instructions is true. I've experienced each one."

Tony came to the table bringing his breath of fresh air attitude along with the breakfast tray. *"Buenos días, amigos."* He smiled as usual. "Hey, Doc, what did you find out? Am I right?"

Doc loved his old buddy. "You're a Mexican Bandito, but yeah you're right. I owe you an ice cream. Cano says it's used for arthritis."

Tony acknowledged me by patting my arm and laughing as only Tony could laugh. "I tried to tell 'em Cano, but you know these old time physicians. Can't tell them anything. If they don't get it in med school, too bad! They just don't get it. My people have known about this treatment for a thousand years!" He stopped his monologue abruptly and just smiled at Jeff, gotcha style.

Jeff acted defeated by hanging his head. He raised his chin and slowly shook his head at the facts. "Amazing! How in hell does the stuff work?"

Tony acted like as though he were bolting out of his chair when he said, "Now he calls it stuff!"

I said, "Well, Doc, first off..."

Doc held up a hand. "Whoa, what are you doing this afternoon around 12:30?"

"Nothing going on in my world."

"Great! How about strolling for a couple? I want and need to know how the clay functions, what it's doing, you know, all the whys and wherefores."

I got it. "For sure Jeff! Be glad to, I'd love to in fact. The clay hasn't been a part of my world for the last year, but I'll answer all of your questions. It's equally simple, complex, and fascinating."

Doug said, "Sounds interesting." For the first time this morning, Doug deliberately placed his fork on his plate, looked directly at me, and asked, "Cano, about the effectiveness of your clay on skin problems. What type specifically are you referring to?"

Doug struck me as a strange mixture of quiet intellect and overt larceny. I knew he must have a good reason for asking a question like that.

"Specifically? Common use you mean? The most notable and effective because it's so widespread, is acne, and I'm not talking about the kids' garden-variety type. I'm talking serious, tough to heal acne."

Doc said, "Really?" He looked at Doug. "Acne's primarily a bacterial infection."

Doug nodded. "Yes I know."

"What we can do with psoriasis has always intrigued me. You

know, the condition is chronic but clay keeps it down and sometimes eradicates it for a long time. The clay is like a miracle to those people."

Together Doc and Doug chimed, "You're kidding?"

I asked, "Why all the questions about dermatology? There are many other uses beside skin treatments."

Doug looked back at me. "What about cancer?"

I raised both my hands. "Frankly, I don't get into that area. I've never had any experience with cancers. I've got some strong beliefs concerning what the clay might do in terms of treating those suffering the effects of chemo, but that's another question."

Doc said, "Cano, have you treated what's called pre-cancerous spots?"

"Yes, those little crusty patches? We've had a lot of luck with them."

Doc said, "Come on!"

"Jeff, I've seen a bunch of 'em in the desert."

Tony grinned and nodded his head like some sort of divine shaman.

Jeff said, "Well I'm not in the desert, but I got one. Been treating it for eighteen months with Retin A."

I was flabbergasted by his admission. "Eighteen months? Too much! Is that the place on your temple? I'm surprised you haven't rubbed the thing off by now."

"Yeah, I know. I keep touching the damn thing."

Tony found an opening. With great pleasure and pride he pointed to Doc. "*Te lo dije!*"

"What'd ya say Tony? Let me in on it!"

"Cano, I said, I told you so. I told these guys that my mother and grandmother used to apply certain clays, *barro*, for things like that."

Ready to leave the table after a good breakfast and interesting discussion, I said,

"Enjoyed it, fellows. I got to do some things and get to work.

Doc, see you at 12:30?"

"Right, and thanks for the info. We've got a lot to discuss."

At 3:00 pm Jeff and I were still walking and talking about Clay Therapy when he said, "Just unbelievable." He stopped and asked, "Cano, have you documented any of what you've told me?"

"Documented? You mean written down? No we were just doing it."

"I know you did it, but no serious sophisticated research and testing ever happened. Right? No record?"

"The only record is in our heads, but it's an ancient therapy. I didn't invent it! Doc, I hope all this talk has filled in some blanks for you, because it sure has rekindled some old fires in me."

"I can imagine. You've got a lot of data flying around in your head. You should get it down on paper."

"At one time I thought about telling the clay therapy story, but I'm not a writer, and doing all this time."

"Maybe that's a plus for you. I've seen some guys do things they didn't think possible."

"You know, lately I've found a reason to consider doing something, but I don't know. Anyway I certainly appreciate this afternoon. It's got me thinking, that's for sure."

Doc laughed. "You appreciate it? Man, I'm the one who really enjoyed it and learned something! I had no idea you had such information and that the stuff would do all this. I mean, now that I see how it works I can also comprehend why it's not marketed extensively." He shook his head in dismay. "It's the crazy state of medicine in this country. Primarily it's because it's not a drug and can't be patented!"

"You got it, Doc, that's it. Besides, it works on far too many different maladies. I agree! It's a crazy world."

Doc absent-mindedly touched the spot on his temple.

I asked, "Doc, what are you thinking?"

My question broke the spell. "Oh, a couple of things." He grew serious and said, "Hell I'm talking to an authority on the subject! I mean it. Cano, you probably know more, have experienced more, than anyone in the country. I believe you've created some tactics and procedures with your clay that might not have been done before."

"I never thought about it like that. I just know what I know, because we did what we did."

He smiled, started to mess with the spot, then conscious of his actions, removed his hand. "You really love the stuff, don't you?"

"Yeah, I guess I do." I hesitated and said, "But…"

"But what?"

" Just that I'm here now with so much time to do. You know, I kinda left it out there."

Jeff said, "That's true, we're here, in prison! I understand. Cano, our cups are full!" A memorable comment from a man doing three life terms. "It's a fact you're here, but it's an open question as to how you do your time. Somehow I don't figure you're going to sit on your butt for the next ten years. No way, I don't see that happening."

"You're right! That's not me I know for sure! In fact, a strange thing happened the other day that's got me thinking about really doing something, but it's just an idea."

Now he had me thinking. "Man if only…"

Jeff jumped into my thought, "If only what?"

"Oh, Doc, I just wish it was here, my clay. I saw this big black guy in our unit with a killer migraine last night. In fact, it damned near put him down. I mean it was driving him crazy."

He said, "Yeah I know. A good man, Big Earl. He has 'em all the time, and you really believe your clay would help a full-blown migraine?"

"Doc, I've never seen a migraine last over forty minutes 'on my skin' as we say here. It has so many uses."

"Tell me about it. There's more need than you realize. Cano, we've got a lot of weird intestinal parasites in here. Nowadays these men come from South America, Africa, Asia. Anyway. I thought the same thing when you mentioned what it'd do as an antibiotic." He was heavy into the idea. "What a coup if we had it here, but the B.O.P., you know, the Bureau of Prisons, will only practice mainstream medicine."

"I understand, Doc. I'll write the idea off and quit dreaming. No chance."

Doc said, "Well, I wouldn't exactly say no chance. I mean, stranger things have happened." He chose his words carefully. "We have a lot of very resourceful people around here."

"Doc, what are you saying?"

"It's shipped in buckets isn't it?"

"Yes, in one and five gallon containers."

"Understand, this place is like a small town. It takes a long list of items to support this prison. We're like an island with special needs and problems of supply to deal with. We have some real talent inside this fence, and problem solving is a major recreation."

I liked the term problem solving. I made a mental note to remember that one.

Jeff continued, "Tony for instance, is a recognized master of importing objects from the real world to the inside. The little guy is resourceful and extremely creative."

I knew Doc McDonald had just told me or at least suggested, an impossible dream.

"Cano, can we use clay for other things that you haven't discussed?"

Doc had me pumped up like a 10-cent balloon. "Oh, hell yes! Several uses. I'll prepare a list!" I was getting ahead of myself. "Doc, do you mean to imply that we can actually do something in here?"

Jeff held up a hand like a school guard. "Hold on! I'm only saying it's a great big wonderful country full of opportunities." His tone told me we had just finished the conversation. "Okay Cano, see you later. I'm gonna do some wind sprints for awhile." We shook hands and he said, "One more issue. I'm curious. Have you discussed your clay with others, inmates I mean?"

"Just off hand. I mean that I had a spa, but nothing in depth like with you guys."

"Good to hear that. I have a hunch you might want to keep the subject private."

"Sure, I have no reason to discuss anything about it."

Jeff grew serious. "Have you ever heard the phrase, *the walls have ears?*"

"Ha! The last time I heard that was when I was a kid in the 40s."

"Well the walls have ears here! Certainly snitches do! Do yourself and me a big favor. Don't discuss your clay or what you know about it with anyone, for any reason! Okay? It's critical to keep this subject private among Doug, Tony, you, and myself as much as possible for now. Remember, loose lips will sink your ship!"

"I understand, Doc. I got it." I felt like I'd been accepted as an integral member of an elite team. I had a brief vision of *Mission Impossible*. I could almost hear the orders of the plot being delivered: "Your mission, if you wish to accept is to..."

Then I thought about "sink your ship" and my heart skipped a beat when I remembered the analogy of the Titanic.

Before I could get entirely carried away, Doc said, "Okay, that's it, thanks for the time and info Cano. See you at chow." We shook hands.

I hardly got out, "All right, Doc, later."

He sprinted away, leaving me with my head spinning and considering what this might all mean. I gathered my wits and began reviewing a few lines of my morning routine "For yesterday is but a dream, tomorrow is only a vision, but today well lived..." I looked up, winked at a big fluffy cloud, inhaled a huge lung full of fresh Oregon air, smiled broadly at the horizon, and took one more lap, a victory lap.

A Resurrection

No man has learned anything until he knows that every day is the judgment day.

Ralph W. Emerson

I came to realize that each thought, silent, audible, bright or dark, is a dedicated prayer, promptly answered and is to the Power what copper wire is to a telephone, stone and steel are to the architect, spring rain is to the wildflower, or new feathers to a young bird.

We can trust the wire to carry the message regardless of the content. We choose the building materials. The spring rain nourishes the flowers and weeds alike. The young bird has the gift of feathers, but still must flap its wings for flight. The Power respects and sustains all living things. The mystical encounter with mother left me rewired and I was ready to go.

Chapter 47

Silent Disciples

In every adversity are the seeds of an equivalent or far greater benefit.
                                                    Ralph Waldo Emerson

A few weeks later, in his usual soft style Tony casually waved as we passed on the compound. "Cano, I need to take a few laps with you. I want to know some things about L.A. Got time?"

Seasoned inmates have a subtle manner of reflecting a message with their eyes when something is important, and he had just told me that something was up.

"Sure, how 'bout this evening?"

"Fine, after chow tonight."

Tony and I enjoyed those laps. Aha! Some stroll indeed. He began with small talk and finally got around to letting me know that our clay had arrived and he had safely tucked it away somewhere inside the razor wire at Sheridan F.C.I.

I couldn't comprehend the news. "Tony, how in hell did you ever get so much clay inside this place?"

Tony stopped dead in his tracks, turned to me and seemed to change into a completely different person when he snapped at me, "Cano, you're new, but not that new! The fact that it's here means that you got what you wanted, and now you have a responsibility to us to use it wisely. We trust you to do what you can do, but understand, how it got here or where it's to be stashed from time to time is no one's business." Then he toned down the lecture. "That's all for your protection."

"Alright, Tony, I understand. Sorry."

"Let me be clear, Cano! Do you recall a brief conversation where not talking about the clay was the subject? The discussion had to do with a corny phrase 'loose lips.' Do you remember?"

I felt like a truant schoolboy. "Yes, I do."

"Good, just so there's no confusion. Loose lips means any needless chatter, any *palabras* about the clay, any talk of any kind, and that includes questions even to me, my friend. Questions mean asking and answering. So any involvement in even a side conversation about the clay must stop. No more! The subject doesn't exist!" He looked at the sky for help. "You held one of those mud wrestling contests! Got it? That's all you know about mud or clay, okay? Is that clear? I mean, to the B.O.P., the stuff is a contraband substance, and that means it's illegal, and that's mucho juicy news for a snitch. And snitches? Cano, let me tell you about these creeps.

"They're a disease around here, they come and go, and we don't always know who they are. Just one rat can bring us down. It could be your cellie. You never know. It could be anyone."

"I'm sorry, Tony, I didn't realize."

"Cano, we know you don't know the ropes, but we do. We'll protect each other by listening and silence. Complete and utter silence gives us our security; that's what we bring to you for your involvement. I might add that we didn't make a final decision until that off-hand remark you made over breakfast about the money."

"The money?"

"Yes the bucks! You said no one was to ever be charged a dime for the your clay. You said that. You still feel the same way?" Tony referred to all the hustles in prison.

"I sure do. I'll never change." I grinned. Tony patted my shoulder, smiled and asked, "What did you people call yourselves out in the desert? The disciples? The Clay Disciples?

Well, my friend," he put his forefinger over his lips and whispered for effect, "Here it will have to be the Silent Disciples."

He paused, and waited for my response. I gave my little mentor a hug. "Thanks, Tony, I'll be careful, but one thing"

"What's that?"

"How can we be sure? I mean when I put the clay on someone or they drink it for whatever reason, how do we know they'll be quiet?"

He looked at me like I was a mystery and said, "You really don't get it do you?" He tried to make me understand. "First off, we'll never have you do your thing unless the hospital can't handle whatever it is or the inmate doesn't want the Administration to know about the problem. You know what I mean?"

"Sure, makes sense, only when there's a real problem. Okay, I got it."

"Cano, listen to me. I can guarantee their silence. I mean, before you ever see them, they'll definitely know what time it is! We'll all know them, but they won't know but a few of us. It would be a silly, foolish, terrible mistake for anyone that we helped to cross us. No! It'll never happen. They'll be 'in' and grateful. I mean they'll owe us. But you're not charging. See what I mean? They'll be told, they'll get it, and they'll respect and protect us." Then as if he was making an understatement on purpose, he hunched over and said, "Oh, yes, they'll be as silent and careful as a little jail house mouse on the razor wire." Tony looked skyward again and with open hands gestured and spoke as if to confirm with the heavens, "Okay? How do you like my speech? I did good, huh?"

He had me gazing at the clouds and smiling in appreciation of his mouse analogy. I liked the name Tony had just popped up with. "Hmmm, the Silent Disciples?" Sounded like the title of a play. Clever. And although it gave me a sense of security, on the other hand with everything being so formalized, I harbored a kind of uneasiness. I wasn't used to so many moving parts that I didn't directly control, but I was in good hands, and a quick learner.

Chapter 48

Mike—From Babe to Man

It is only the wisest and the very stupidest who can not change.

Confucius

In the early 90s, Sheridan F.C.I. had a large and interesting population of pot growers and bank robbers. Although opposites in substance and style, each group represented a specialized type of labor, producing volumes of unique and delightful stories.

The genuine affection and respect for my lady from so many in prison, validated her integrity and was a humbling satisfaction to me. All because of the Silent Disciples.

In prison, I learned very quickly to discriminate who I associated with. Inmates don't care to be seen in trashy company, including who they speak to and who they sit with at meals. Needless to say, I didn't encourage thieves, such as most criminal lawyers, to tell their story. As a rule their larceny proves far too much to hold down on an empty stomach.

If the potential meal mate qualified in either field, say bank robber or pot grower, I often asked them to have a seat and then followed that with, "Would you consider telling me a story? You know, about your work?"

They usually responded with, "Are you serious?"

"As a matter of fact I really am, I mean if you don't mind. My name is Cano Graham." I'd offer my hand and the guest would politely respond before thinking too much, and we would proceed.

My invitee on one particular morning was a sharp featured, twenty-five year old Yaqui Indian from Sonora, Mexico and southern Texas. I later learned he had been hooked on heroin since the age of fourteen. Because of a Yaqui name that no one could pronounce, everyone called him Mike. Everyone considered him a bit strange because he never discussed his childhood or anything considered personal. Mike was a walking enigma. The inmate population was well aware that Mike was a dedicated pro in his chosen profession, bank robbery. He had long ago achieved celebrity status for his imaginative and daring nineteen on-the-job training episodes. He succeeded eighteen times. Tough trade! You only have to be fouled one time to lose the entire game.

Mike had been down and clean for six years when I met him, and he still hadn't cut that pure black hair. He leaned back, and with good humor pointed a plastic fork at me and said, "Now I know who you are! You're the guy that's into stories. Yeah, I've heard of you. Tony told me about you-hmmm." He hesitated then smiled. "Well, once upon a time." He laughed in the wonderful natural way that Indians all seem to have, and said, "Sorry to say, Mr. Cano, but this little story ended up on the front page of the San Diego, California newspaper." After a slight pause he said, "It also got me twenty years."

"Really? Twenty years? Be my guest. Go right ahead. Sounds like a dandy!"

"Oh, it's a dandy all right!" He reflected for a moment, set his fork down, looked me straight in the eyes, slightly moved his head in wonder and said thoughtfully, "I was a mighty sick kid. The smack had me all tied up." He looked at me as though he wondered if I truly understood where he was coming from. He went ahead, "Mr. Cano, I didn't know any other way to go. By then the stuff was all I knew or cared about."

"I got it. Hey, Mike, I haven't been there, but I can relate to a degree."

Mike smiled, nodded slightly. "So a story, huh? Are you a writer, Mr. Cano?"

"Oh, no, I just find stories about real people interesting."

He nodded again. "I believe you do."

I had a serious, bright, and complex individual in front of me. His impeccable table manners told me that someone had raised him properly. What happened I did not know. His mystery lay hidden in his early childhood. I'd get to it another time. For the time being I had to stay with what I had.

I said, "I mean, if you feel up to it, I'd be interested in hearing about it."

"Sure, it'll do me good this morning to remember where I came from."

I thought that statement alone was a hell of a thing for a young man to say. Just as he began to say something, Mike bit into some crisp bacon, flinched painfully, and held his jaw. "Damn!" He got up from the table and through clenched teeth said, "Will you excuse me a minute?"

He went to a trashcan, spit blood, returned and said, "I've got a bad tooth. It's abscessed." He made no other mention of the pain, and continued our conversation. He poured lots of cream and seven packs of sugar into his coffee, and then tasted a spoonful to make sure it was perfect. "All right, first off you've got to have a plan." He leaned forward and said, "Not just an idea, but a complete plan. Got it?"

"Ah, yeah, I understand. A plan. Go ahead."

Without further discussion, Mike began to recount and relive his last day in the free world. The seething emotion of the bizarre episode was enhanced not merely by moving dialogue, but through the quickening and tone of his voice, all accentuated by deep, soulful, brown eyes. He was there again, but this morning as a spectator rather than a participant. Mike was physically present, but it was as though he was plunging back into the past life of a long departed brother.

Mike began to take on a different persona, and he took me along. "The bank was close to downtown San Diego. I decided to hit it on a bicycle."

"A bicycle?"

"Mr. Cano, you've got to understand. I had reasons. I could disappear quicker on a bike than in a car."

"Oh?" His logic intrigued me.

"Oh, yes! A lot quicker. I could turn a corner and ditch the bike in a second."

"Really?" I had trouble picturing the scene.

"Besides that, my pickup wasn't in the best shape. In fact, it wasn't running at the time, but it didn't matter, the bike was fine. I'd nabbed it the night before. The thing was like brand new. One of those ten-speed, fancy jobs, you know?"

"I don't ride bikes."

"Too bad! Good exercise. You're missing something. Anyway, so I'm all set." He became demonstrative again. "I peddled up to the bank parking lot. I had my backpack on and I parked my bike just like a regular customer. As soon as I got inside I looked around to check on things."

"Excuse me again Mike, but was your hair the same length as now?"

"My hair? Sure, same as now, like always. I never cut it. Why?"

"Just wondering how you appeared at the time."

"Like now. Normal."

At first I thought he was kidding. He wasn't. In his mind he was a normal looking citizen. I got ahead of myself and imagined the coming scene. His attention generating pure black, waist-length hair was flying carefree behind him while he had a backpack of the bank's money and peddling peacefully on a new ten speed stolen bike. Classic. "So I entered the teller's line that looked *right.* You know what I mean?"

"I can imagine the scene."

He began to internalize his delivery again, only now more so. "She was an elderly, big white lady, must have been forty-five to fifty years old."

I cracked a smile at his interpretation of old but drew it back before he noticed.

Caught up in his memory, Mike had stopped eating. "When I got to the counter I handed her a note to fill up my paper sack. Now, Mr. Cano, this is the critical time. If they get too scared they'll freeze up or worse, they'll yell! That's the bad news 'cause it spooks everyone, and a fella doesn't know what to do. Still and all I had to let her know I was serious, you know what I mean?" Mike said that a lot. "Anyway she read the note and just stared at me, blank like."

I thought, what a sight for this lady. I could just hear her relating what she saw.

Mike said, "I had to take control, so I said firmly, Fill up the sack! Fast! And no dye packs!"

"That must be exciting! I mean to actually do it"

"Tell me about it! Mr. Cano, it's a real rush."

He had me on the edge of my chair. "So? What happened next?"

Mike increased the tempo. "For a fat lady she moved fast, and in a quick minute handed me the grocery bag of money. I calmly placed it in my backpack and strolled real cool-like out of the bank."

"Damn, Mike, you did it!"

"Yeah, I was out of the bank, on my bike and rolling when my world fell apart. I was two full blocks away, with every thing going smooth as silk, when a dye pack went off, sounding like slapping a feather pillow. You know?" His hands flew out and up. "Poof! And this cloud of red dye smoke was pouring out of my backpack like I was a plane on fire. Hell, Mr. Cano, I was on a main street in sunny downtown San Diego!" The drama had evolved into a

383

serious comedy.

"Mike, what in the world did you do? I mean, my God, what a place to be!"

He laughed at the memory. "Aw, I kinda lost it. You know what I mean? Everything had been going just as planned. I really needed the money. I mean I was sick. I needed my medicine. Plus my truck needing brakes, and tires and all."

"What did you do when you saw the dye?"

"I'll tell you what I did! I emptied the backpack of dyed money. I threw the whole paper bag into a trash bin, went back to the same bank, walked up to the old fat lady and said, I told you, 'No dye packs! I told you that! And you broke your word! Now do it again! And no tricks or I'm gonna get really mad. Do it!"

"You didn't! Tell me you're kidding."

"Nope. I got clean away again, with a sack of good money!"

I held my head in disbelief.

"Didn't make it though! They grabbed me a couple of blocks away, a traffic cop at that. Can you imagine?"

I could only shake my head in awe.

"I guess it didn't take Sherlock Holmes to locate me." By now he had lightened up somewhat, and laughed at himself. "Whew! Mr. Cano, I tell you this, it all seems more like a dream than real!" He glanced around the chow hall and said, "But I'm here, and that's no dream. And now I'm clean!" He smiled and said, "That's a dream I never thought I'd experience. I'm a lucky man, you know what I mean?"

I nodded. I got it. "Yes, you are Mike, lucky indeed."

"Who's lucky?" The question came from Tony as he set his breakfast tray down on the table. "Morning, gents."

"Hey, Tony! Mike here's telling me a hell of a tale."

Tony looked at Mike and back to me, "Mike told you one of his stories? I'll be. You don't say. That's a first."

"Yes, he did, and a heck of a story at that."

Mike smiled broadly. "Tony, I told Mr. Cano about the last

one."

Tony was surprised. "About the dye pack and bicycle? No, come on, really?"

Mike was still nodding. "Yes."

Tony started eating, "What a way to begin a day. Will wonders never cease?"

I didn't understand his comment.

Tony looked at my guest and said, "Mike, have you ever told that story outside of our NA (narcotics anonymous) meetings. Ever?"

Mike shyly shook his head. "No I haven't! It just seemed okay to tell Mr. Cano this morning."

Tony was enjoying all this. "I'm glad you did, proud of you, boy!" He looked at me and confirmed what I was thinking. "Mike's a much different man today, wouldn't you agree, Cano?"

"To say the least. Wow! Looks like our Mike has become a man. That story was about another person."

Tony agreed. "No question about it. Our friend is a good man with a fine mind. He has a great future when he gets out of here."

Mike interrupted, raised a finger and said, "One correction, please." He smiled and said, "I have a future today, and every day, and not just when I get out of here."

Tony looked at me proudly. "Out of the mouths of babes."

I pushed away from the table, stood up, placed a hand on Mike's shoulder, and said, "This babe has become a man, for real." While I stood, I remembered a thought by Shakespeare. *They say, best men are molded out of faults, and for the most, become much more the better for being a little bad.*

Then to Mike, in a way that let him know he had a solid new friend I said, "Thanks, Mike, you just made my day. See you around."

Afterword

The next ten years in Sheridan, Oregon FCI and Bastrop, Texas FCI, proved to be the most productive chapter of my life. Though not by choice, my energy was harnessed, my aspiration focused. The many inmates involved held their secret as a private possession, that of sharing the highest respect for the healing power of the clay.

I accept their appreciation on my lady's behalf, and must add that this validation comes from some of the finest people, the inmates. They have some of the most inspiring and dramatic episodes of healing. Theirs is a separate book, *The Silent Disciples*, to be released in 2007.

Once upon a time, I knew nothing about clay, neither its existence, nor its uses. However, my stay in Tecopa Hot Springs changed all that, and gave me a mission in life: to give people the knowledge of using clay therapeutically to help them heal themselves. That is what this book and my life are all about.

I have included many of the stories of the people I have known over the years, and their experiences with the clay; however, I found it impossible to include all of them. So, I have saved them to populate another book.

Yes, it's different, this new affection for clay. The ancient survival technique of utilizing clay to detox, and protect the system, allowing the body to heal itself, is simple and natural, almost instinctive; as if the body and the clay had always been kindred spirits. After all, she's the stuff we're made of.

As always, I wish you health and happiness,

Cano Graham

The Clay Disciples
Healing Archives

Our Mission:

to educate and research

We have created an ever-expanding, full-spectrum, online library of pertinent clay information. You may access that information by going to: www.globalclayresearch.com. Because the uses of clay are many and varied, I have put together an ebook that will give you the details of methods and therapies to help heal a number of maladies. I've chosen the ebook format for this because it will make a much more efficient resource for your needs.

Prerequisite for Healing/Detoxing

Clay therapy has been with us for millennia. Since the first of our kind walked the earth, clay has held an important place in man's healing history. Volumes of oral and written material has made its way into medical archives, but for a very long time, no one knew why it worked, they only knew that it healed.

Truth be known, the clay itself does not heal; it does, however, act as Nature's ultimate healing catalyst, nourishing and cleansing and *making conditions right for the body to heal itself.* Over the years, we have discovered three fundamental and powerful facts about using clay therapeutically as an antibiotic, detoxing agent, and circulation enhancer.

1-Certain clays act as powerful antibiotics and wound healers. The clay seeks out and kills the infecting bacteria and speeds the healing process.

2-Certain clays act as powerful detoxing agents. Heavy metals, chemicals, and toxins are all positively charged and are irresistibly attracted to the clay.

3-The action of clay dramatically stimulates the body's blood circulation. The result completes the debris evacuation process and *allows the body to heal itself.*

With these facts in mind, consider the following partial list of uses for clay therapy.

Prevention or Treatment of Diseases and other Conditions

Mouth: oral hygiene, gum disease, abscesses, sores.

Stomach: ulcer, dyspepsia, acid reflux, food poisoning.

Colon care: hemorrhoid, fistula

Skin care: clay mask, shingles, rashes, psoriasis, acne, rosacea, eczema, fungus, (body, nails).

Stops bleeding and speeds healing.

Wound healing: laceration, abrasions, blisters, burns.

Pain: arthritis, migraine, analgesic

Sports: sprain, bruise, shinsplints, sore feet.

Stress Reduction

Women's issues: yeast infection, chlamydia, bladder infection, vaginal fistula, menopause, bacterial vaginosis, PMS, PPS, pregnancy, milk duct infections, stretch marks.

Insect/animal bites: scorpion, brown recluse, fire ants, spiders, mosquitoes.

SPECIAL RESEARCH CONSIDERATION: post polio syndrome, prostate problems, chemical poisoning, Lyme disease, sepsis, ear infection, diabetic legs and feet, symptoms of HIV/AIDS.

ACKNOWLEDGEMENT

In my inaugural edition of *The Clay Disciples*, I recognize Jason Eyton (www.eytonsearth.org) to be among the quintessential pioneers of the contemporary movement of clay therapy.

The Love Child

All the world knows me in my book and my book in me.
Michel Montagne

In 1987 I had an absolutely mad affair with a lovely lady, a free spirit from Tecopa Hot Springs, California. This relationship resulted in the birth of a child. I had always wanted a son, but fortunately, destiny in her wisdom blessed me with a beautiful daughter.

In retrospect, I realize she came along at just the right time. Good things seem to do that. When she came into my life I was physically lonely, mentally stagnant, and emotionally scattered. I was going one hundred miles per-hour, spinning my wheels like the proverbial hamster in a cage. On the surface, my life flowed smoothly, but it was only an illusion.

My child's birth calmed my troubled spirit, roused intense fatherly instincts I didn't even know I had, and filled my days with gratitude for her existence. It was impossible to stay submerged in my own adverse circumstances as long as I kept myself busy nurturing my precious daughter. She came late in my life, but nothing could deter me from creating a life for my baby.

The Child's mother, a recognized Healer, commanded great respect, but as I have mentioned before, she was also a free spirit, belonging to no one. So the job of parenting rested squarely on my willing shoulders. My precocious youngster kept me busy and jumping. First, by not allowing her to be taken away, and second by keeping her going in the right direction. She takes after her mother in many ways, so I had to be careful not to interfere too much with her independent nature. After the normal episodes and challenges associated with growth, the daily pages and chapters of this young girl's life accumulated.

All these years later, it thrills me to say that she is now entering a terrific position in the literary world. Her publisher felt she needed to have some rough edges trimmed before turning her loose, but I'm kind of fond of those edges.

I had mixed emotions about all of this refinement and dressing-up business that she had to go through, but I shouldn't worry so much. From the first moment I helped my baby stand on her own, she has been walking and taking her own space. She is not timid or weak, and she no longer needs me to defend her. However, it can be a rough and tumble world where she is going. She is not as polished or politically correct as some of her peers, but she is real, and will be known as a get-it-done, hard-driving worker. It's time for her to stretch her wings and prove herself.

I'm still not used to the idea that she doesn't need me anymore, and I'm sad that she's gone. She grew up so fast!

Her mother and I enjoyed a few short years together before I had to go away for a long time. Fortunately, I was able to keep my child close by. Time passed so quickly, as my own mother assured me that it would.

I hope you've enjoyed meeting my love child. You've just read her last page. Oh, I know you've already guessed this, but my child's mother was none other than my lady, the clay, and my love child's name? She is affectionately called The Clay Disciples. She loves you.

Good luck. Good health. Go easy, friend.

Cano Graham

Acknowledgements

I wish thank Joan Neubauer of *WordWright.biz* for her professional editing, Joseph Youmans for his creative support and friendship over the years, and Mickie Phipps for her friendship and critical input in the final editing process.

To discover more go to www.globalclayresearch.com

This website will provide you with current and updated information on where to order clay or how to purchase additional copies of *The Clay Disciples.* You can get answers to your questions about clay and you can also contact Cano Graham.

Dental
P. 55
76
80
82
144
381

Feet
P. 78

Arm
P. 87

Foot
P. 96

(chemical sensitivity sores)
P 178

RSI
Finger injury video player P. 262

migraine
P 239-244   scorpion bite
95-6   P. 134-42
               ulcers
                  P. 147-8

Arthritis on leknader
   P. 165-6

Shingles   skin
              fungus
      P. 233-238

PMS
P. 159 -61

leg ulcer/ gangrene
152-4,
sprained ankle
   P. 230-232

Rectal fistula
   P. 154

Bentonite Clay   Pelotherapy
P. 90
P. 92
P. 98   RAYMOND DEXTREIT French

Toxic Shock Syndrome
   P 195-201

Road accident
P 214-9
Arthritis p 211

P. 126 P. 125
arthritis splint in finger

Shingles   Head wound
           P. 110
p 237-8

Multiple Chemical Sensitivity
   P. 203 -

P. 144 Food poisoning

steam burn   kreosote burn
   P 205- 210   P. 220-23

Printed in the United States
205064BV00002B/189/A